D1590564

Colombo's
Tips & Tricks
with
Drug-Eluting Stents

This Book is dedicated to all the Fellows who have been and who are working in Columbus and San Raffaele Hospitals

Colombo's Tips & Tricks with Drug-Eluting Stents

Edited by

Antonio Colombo MD
EMO Centro Cuore Columbus, Milan
and
San Raffaele Hospital
Milan, Italy

and

Goran Stankovic MD
Institute for Cardiovascular Diseases
Clinical Center of Serbia
Belgrade
Serbia and Montenegro

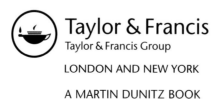

Taylor & Francis
Taylor & Francis Group

LONDON AND NEW YORK

A MARTIN DUNITZ BOOK

© 2005 Taylor & Francis, an imprint of the Taylor & Francis Group

First published in the United Kingdom in 2005
by Taylor & Francis,
an imprint of the Taylor & Francis Group,
2 Park Square, Milton Park
Abingdon, Oxon OX14 4RN

Tel.:   +44 (0)20 7017 6000
Fax.:   +44 (0)20 7017 6699
Website: www.tandf.co.uk

All rights reserved. No part of this publication may be reproduced, stored in a retrieval system, or transmitted, in any form or by any means, electronic, mechanical, photocopying, recording, or otherwise, without the prior permission of the publisher or in accordance with the provisions of the Copyright, Designs and Patents Act 1988 or under the terms of any licence permitting limited copying issued by the Copyright Licensing Agency, 90 Tottenham Court Road, London W1P 0LP.

Although every effort has been made to ensure that all owners of copyright material have been acknowledged in this publication, we would be glad to acknowledge in subsequent reprints or editions any omissions brought to our attention.

British Library Cataloguing in Publication Data

Data available on application

Library of Congress Cataloging-in-Publication Data

Data available on application

ISBN 1-84184-396-2

Distributed in North and South America by

Taylor & Francis
2000 NW Corporate Blvd
Boca Raton, FL 33431, USA

Within Continental USA
Tel.: 800 272 7737; Fax.: 800 374 3401
Outside Continental USA
Tel.: 561 994 0555; Fax.: 561 361 6018
E-mail: orders@crcpress.com

Distributed in the rest of the world by
Thomson Publishing Services
Cheriton House
North Way
Andover, Hampshire SP10 5BE, UK
Tel.: +44 (0) 1264 332424
E-mail: salesorder.tandf@thomsonpublishingservices.co.uk

Composition by Siva Math Setters, Chennai, India
Printed and bound by Scotprint, Haddington, UK

Contents

The text of this book is to be used in conjunction with the two CD-ROMs that accompany it. All references in the book to slides, frames etc. that are printed in blue are references to PowerPoint format images supplied on the CD-ROMs. Chapters 1–6 are on CD 1 and chapters 7–10 and the index are on CD 2. In addition, the entire book is included in Acrobat PDF format. Please refer to page xvii for further information on how to use the CD-ROMs.

Preface

The introduction of drug-eluting stents represents a major landmark in cardiovascular medicine because it offers the possibility of shifting the mode of treatment of ischemic heart disease towards percutaneous intervention.

This fact represents a historical milestone: 'restenosis has been conquered after more than a decade of siege'.

The pleasure in writing about the usage of drug-eluting stents is enormous because for the first time we are able to experience the feeling that what we are doing will most likely continue for some time to come.

As Dr Paul Teirstein wrote, 'it is a nice feeling for a surgeon to realize that the gallbladder he just removed will not grow back again', and we are now experiencing the same feeling when we place a drug-eluting stent in a stenosis and we are able to see the final result and know that this result will stay as it is for a long period of time.

Technical changes brought about by the introduction of drug-eluting stents are enormous. The most important and fundamental of these is that we are not afraid to implant a long stent. In the early days of coronary stenting I made a presentation that stated that a stent is a prosthesis and needs to be anchored on healthy tissue (vessel). This statement introduced the concept of stenting from healthy to healthy. Unfortunately the appearance of diffuse in-stent restenosis quickly demanded a revision of this approach to one of full lesion coverage. Under some criticism, we tried to introduce the technique of spot stenting: a laborious, time-consuming and sometimes uncertain approach. No more spot stenting, or as Dr Marty Leon remarked: 'Antonio you should "stent every spot"'. We are delighted we can 'stent every spot' and that we can go back to the concept of full lesion coverage.

The philosophy of this book and the CDs that accompany it, is to convey most of the new technical elements brought into play by the usage of drug-eluting stents and by their different performance characteristics. The concepts expressed are a clear departure from our prior work *Tips & Tricks in Interventional Cardiology*. The emphasis now is to be able to treat most, if not all, the clinically relevant lesions. We are no longer afraid of diffuse disease, small vessels or bifurcations; we now feel more secure when treating unprotected left main lesions. We have tried to give more emphasis to detailed description of cases and to summarize in a simple message the most relevant teaching points. As usual, we unfortunately have a section about complications and problems, a section which perhaps one day will cease to exist. Nevertheless, this section is a little smaller than in the past, with coronary perforations and ruptures being the main representatives. An important message to the industry is for it to provide the interventional cardiologist with better tools with which to treat these types of complications.

Compared with our previous publication, we now have additional co-authors, all of whom have done an excellent and timely job and I would like to thank them again.

Dr Goran Stankovic has been responsible for pushing me to undertake this second project and as a 'punishment' he has had to contend with a year of intense work to help with all the editing. This book would have never been completed without Goran's support. Giovanni Martini also requires specific recognition for all his superb skills in putting together the images and videos, that are so important in this type of presentation. Finally, special thanks to Alan Burgess at Martin Dunitz who made this publication possible and was instrumental in the introduction of a number of helpful new features.

Antonio Colombo MD

List of contributors

Alaide Chieffo MD
San Raffaele Hospital
Università Vita Salute
via Olgettina 60
20132 Milan
Italy

David J Cohen MD MSc
Cardiovascular Division
Beth Israel Deaconess Medical Center
330 Brookline Avenue
Boston, MA 02215
USA

Antonio Colombo MD
EMO Centro Cuore Columbus
via M. Buonarroti 48
20145 Milan
and
San Raffaele Hospital
Università Vita Salute
via Olgettina 60
20132 Milan
Italy

Keith D Dawkins MD
Wessex Cardiac Unit
Southampton University
Mail Point 46
Tremona Road, E. Level East Wing
Southampton SO16 6YD
UK

Dan Greenberg PhD
Cardiovascular Division
Beth Israel Deaconess Medical
    Center
330 Brookline Avenue
Boston, MA 02215
USA

Ioannis Iakovou MD
EMO Centro Cuore Columbus
via M. Buonarroti 48
20145 Milan
Italy

Giovanni Martini RT
EMO Centro Cuore Columbus
via M. Buonarroti 48
20145 Milan
Italy

Kazuaki Mitsudo MD
Kurashiki Central Hospital
1-1-1 Miwa Kurashiki
Okayama 710-8602
Japan

Jeffrey W Moses MD
Columbia University Medical Center
161 Fort Washington Avenue
New York, NY 10032
USA

Issam Moussa MD
Columbia University Medical Center
161 Fort Washington Avenue
New York, NY 10032
USA

John Ormiston MD
Mercy Angiography, PO Box 9911
Newmarket
Auckland
New Zealand

Miodrag Ostojic MD
Institute for Cardiovascular Diseases
Clinical Center of Serbia
Koste Todorovica 8
11000 Belgrade
Serbia and Montenegro

Eugenio Picano MD
Consiglio Nazionale delle Ricerche
Institute of Clinical Physiology
via Moruzzi 1
56124 Pisa
Italy

Matthew J Price MD
Division of Cardiovascular Diseases
Scripps Clinic and Research
    Foundation
10666 North Torrey Pines Road
La Jolla, CA 92037-8411
USA

Goran Stankovic MD
Institute for Cardiovascular Diseases
Clinical Center of Serbia
Koste Todorovica 8
11000 Belgrade
Serbia and Montenegro

Paul S Teirstein MD
Division of Cardiovascular Diseases
Scripps Clinic and Research
    Foundation
10666 North Torrey Pines Road
La Jolla, CA 92037-8411
USA

Vladan Vukcevic MD
Institute for Cardiovascular Diseases
Clinical Center of Serbia
Koste Todorovica 8
11000 Belgrade
Serbia and Montenegro

Giora Weisz MD
Columbia University Medical Center
161 Fort Washington Avenue
New York, NY 10032
USA

How to use the CD-ROMs

GETTING STARTED

- Save your work and quit all programs that are running on your computer.
- Place one of the CD-ROMs onto the opened CD-ROM drawer and close.
- The CD-ROM will automatically begin.
- If your computer is running slowly or experiencing problems, then you should eject the CD-ROM and re-start your computer. Then follow the above steps again.
- There are two CD-ROMs: CD 1 contains chapters 1–6, and CD 2 chapters 7–10.

Minimum Computer Specifications

PC
- Intel Processor (Pentium IV) or equivalent
- 128 MB RAM
- 16 bit color
- 1024 × 768 display
- 16× CD-ROM
- Windows 98/ME/2000/XP

Apple Macintosh
- 128 MB RAM (free)
- 16 bit color
- 1024 × 768 display
- 16× CD-ROM
- OS X

Introduction

These CD-ROMs contain a wealth of information which can all be accessed through the menu on the left of the computer screen. Double-click folders to open them and single-click the files within them. You will find PowerPoint presentations of each topic and a copy of the book in Acrobat PDF format on the disk.

Essentially these disks allow you to browse through the PowerPoint files and the electronic version (PDF) of the book to find exactly what you are looking for. If you want to edit the PowerPoint presentations, you can save them to your hard drive in the location of your choice and then open them in PowerPoint on your computer. If you have any problems, you can refer to the Help pages for information on how to use the CD-ROMs.

The 'Read-Me' documentation on CD1 contains information to help start the CD-ROMs and provides trouble-shooting advice.

Main Menu

The main menu is on the left side of the computer screen. It is organized into a tree structure that allows a familiar way of accessing the information on the disk. You will find that as you access different folders, the interface will adapt to allow you to manipulate the information.

You can use your mouse to drop down folders and select sub items. Note that there are also commonly used keyboard shortcuts to do this. Use your arrow keys to navigate up and down the list, and hit the spacebar to open a folder that you have selected. Hitting the spacebar a second time will close the folder again. You can achieve the same results by using the left and right arrow keys. Hitting a key on your keyboard that matches with the first letter of a currently available menu item will result in the next item in the list, starting with that letter or number, being highlighted.

In almost all folders, apart from the Introduction you will be given options to either go to the relevant page in the book, or to launch the PowerPoint slide show associated with that section of the book.

Book and PDF Controls

When viewing the book, you will see a screen displaying an Acrobat PDF copy of book in the main viewable area in the middle of the screen. In the top menu bar, there is a search facility, and in the bottom menu bar, the PDF controls for the book.

With the search bar you can enter a word or phrase and click 'Search'. This will search through the book for the first available instance of the search text. Clicking the 'Search' button again, consecutively searches for other instances of the text throughout the book until no further occurrences are found.

The PDF control bar allows you to browse through the book, select text, and print out ranges of pages of the book or the entire book. You can also use the standard 'page up' and 'page down' to scroll up and down through the book.

Links

You will find that references to slides, frames and runs (video clips) are colored blue in the book text. References are colored pink. Single-clicking on the blue links will take you to the relevant PowerPoint slide or video clip and single-clicking on a pink link will take you to the relevant reference at the PubMed website if you are connected to the Internet.

PowerPoint Presentations

The main tree menu on the left of the screen allows you to select from the disk and launch the various PowerPoint presentations associated with each chapter. When you click on one of the PowerPoint slide show options from the menu, the copy of PowerPoint that is installed on your own computer will be launched to show you the presentation. From here you can use standard PowerPoint controls to view the presentation. If you do not have a copy of PowerPoint installed, then you will not be able to view the presentations.

When exiting a PowerPoint presentation, you will also notice a message in the middle of the screen advising you that there may be additional material associated with the presentation. These might be, for example, JPEG images which you can now view by clicking 'Browse'.

1

Drug-Eluting Stent Platforms

Sirolimus-eluting stents: from clinical trials to real world

Alaide Chieffo MD

Over the past decade, the use of bare-metal stents (BMS) has become common practice during percutaneous coronary intervention (PCI). Although stents significantly reduce restenosis when compared with balloon angioplasty, restenosis rates in patients who receive stents are still 20–40% at 6 months.[1,2] Recently, the concept of using stents coated with agents that could potentially inhibit neointimal hyperplasia has emerged, and drug-eluting stents (DES) represent one of the fastest growing fields in interventional cardiology today.

Sirolimus is a potent antiproliferative and immunosuppressive agent which binds the cytosolic receptor FKBP12 and blocks an enzyme-denominated TOR-kinase (target of sirolimus), upregulating p27 levels and therefore inhibiting the phosphorylation of retinoblastoma protein (pRb) with blockage of the cell cycle progression at the G1-S transition (slide 1).[3]

Preliminary studies with sirolimus-eluting stents (SES) showed encouraging results regarding the efficacy of these stents in preventing in-stent restenosis. The sirolimus-coated Bx Velocity stent (Cordis) is fabricated from medical 316 LS stainless steel. It is available in two cell configurations (six-cell configuration: expanded diameter 2.5–3.25 mm) and seven-cell design (expanded diameter 3.5–3.75 mm). The stent contains $140\,\mu g$ rapamycin/cm^2, which gives a total rapamycin content of $153\,\mu g$ on the six-cell stent and $180\,\mu g$ on the seven-cell stent. The coating formulation consists of 30% rapamycin by weight in a 50 : 50 mixture of the polymers polyethylenevinyl-acetate (PEVA) and polybutylmethacrylate (PBMA).[4]

The First In Man (FIM) study was the first published nonrandomized study in humans to investigate stents coated with antimitotic agents (slides 2–4).[5] It was conducted to assess the efficacy of sirolimus-eluting stents (SES) in inhibiting neointimal hyperplasia. In the FIM study, two different formulations of SES were evaluated: fast release ($n=15$) and slow release ($n=30$). This study, initially performed in São Paulo and then extended to Rotterdam, enrolled 45 patients, the first 15 of whom were treated with fast-release (FR) drug-eluting stent (GI), with the slow-release (SR) drug-eluting stent being given to the following 30 patients (GII in São Paulo and GIII in Rotterdam). Virtual absence of neointimal proliferation was documented by serial intravascular ultrasound (IVUS) and angiography at all time points (4, 6, 12, and 24 months) in both groups.[5–7] One patient had target-vessel

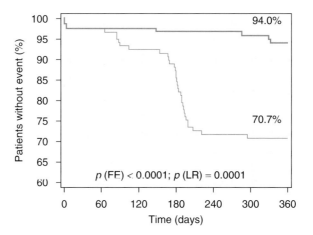

Figure 1   RAVEL event-free survival: death, MI, CABG, re-PTCA

thrombosis at 14 months. There was no in-stent restenosis (ISR) up to 2 years, and the overall major adverse cardiac event (MACE) rate was 11.1%, including procedural complications. No death occurred after hospital discharge. This pioneer investigation provides unique long-term data on sirolimus-eluting stents and allays some of the concerns about a potential late 'catch-up' of restenosis or late side effects.

'The RAndomized study with the Sirolimus-coated Bx VELocity balloon expandable stent in the treatment of patients with *de novo* native coronary artery lesions' the (RAVEL) study[8,9] was the first randomized trial to compare slow-release SES with bare Bx Velocity stents in single, *de novo* lesions in native coronary arteries (slides 5–7, Figure 1). Patients (238) were randomized to receive either a SES ($n = 120$) or an uncoated stent ($n = 118$). At 6 months, the unique result of 0% angiographic restenosis and a mean in-stent late loss (LL) of −0.01 for the group treated with SES was achieved. In the SES group, cumulative event-free survival was 94.2 and 89.2% at 1 and 2 years, respectively vs. 70.7 and 70.3% in the control group (all revascularizations were included). In the RAVEL study, 44 patients were diabetic; 19 received SES and 25 were treated with BMS.[10] There was zero restenosis in the SES groups (diabetic and non-diabetic) compared with a 42% rate in the diabetic population assigned to bare-metal stents ($p = 0.001$). After 12 months, the event-free survival rate was 90% in the SES vs. 52% in the control group ($p < 0.01$). There were no target-lesion revascularizations (TLRs) in either SES group compared with a 36% rate in the diabetic bare-metal stent group ($p = 0.007$).

These initial studies included small numbers of patients, with relatively simple coronary lesions. More recently, the 'SIRolImUS-coated Bx Velocity stent in the treatment of patients with *de novo* coronary artery lesions' the (SIRIUS),[11] and the 'European-SIRIUS' (E-SIRIUS)[12] trials included patients at a higher risk of restenosis (more diabetic patients, longer lesions, and smaller vessels).

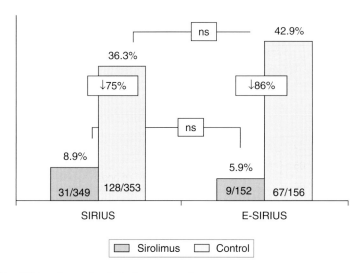

Figure 2   QCA at 8 months: In-lesion restenosis

The SIRIUS trial[11] was a randomized, double-blind trial, which enrolled 1058 patients, with a lesion length between 15 and 30 mm, randomly assigned to receive a standard stent or a SES. SES (Cypher, Cordis) contained 140 µg of sirolimus per cm^2 embedded in a copolymer matrix 5–10 µm thick, designed to release 80% of the drug in 30 days (slides 7–17, Figure 2). The primary end-point of target-vessel failure (TVF), defined as the composite end-point of death from cardiac causes, myocardial infarction (Q wave or non-Q wave), and target-vessel revascularization (TVR), occurred in 46 patients (8.6%) in the SES group vs. 110 patients (21%) in the BMS group, with a 58% relative reduction ($p < 0.001$). There were no acute stent thromboses, one case of subacute stent thrombosis occurred in each group, and there were four late stent thromboses (one in the SES and three in the BMS). The cumulative frequency of thrombosis was similar in the two groups (0.4% in SES vs. 0.8% in BMS). At angiographic follow-up, late lumen loss was improved in SES (0.17 and 0.24 mm, respectively, vs. 1.00 and 0.81 mm in BMS; $p < 0.001$ for all comparisons). Similarly, there was a reduction in restenosis rate, in-stent as well as in-segment, in SES (3.2 and 8.9%) compared with standard stent (35.4 and 36.3%) ($p < 0.001$ for both comparisons). Intravascular ultrasound (IVUS) sub-analysis showed that this reduction was obtained mainly through a reduction of neointimal hyperplasia volume, from 57.6 to 4 mm^3 ($p < 0.001$).

Important subgroup analyses conducted in the SIRIUS trial showed a sustained benefit of SES over BMS across specific subsets of complex lesions or patients: diabetic patients (50.5 vs. 17.6% in-segment restenosis, and 22.3 vs. 6.9% in TLR); and lesions located in small vessels (42.9 vs. 18.4% in-segment restenosis, and 20.6 vs. 7.3% in TLR). In addition to the reduction of overall angiographic restenosis, an

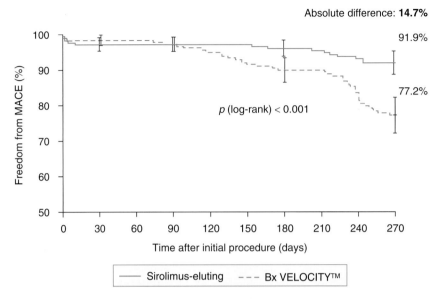

Figure 3   E-SIRIUS: 9-month survival: free from MACE

important finding of the SIRIUS study was also a change in the pattern of restenosis, with a reduction in the rate of diffuse pattern (restenotic lesion >10 mm in length) from 58 to 13% ($p<0.001$), respectively, in the standard stent and SES. At 12 months, the absolute difference in TLR continued to increase and was 4.9% in SES vs. 20% in TLR ($p<0.001$). There were no differences in death or myocardial infarction (MI) rates. In high-risk patient subsets, defined by vessel size, lesion length, and presence of diabetes mellitus, there was a 70–80% reduction in clinical restenosis at 1 year.[13]

In the E-SIRIUS study,[12] 352 patients, with smaller vessels (2.5–3.0 mm) and longer lesions (15–32 mm) compared with the SIRIUS trial,[11] were randomized to receive SES vs. BMS (slides 17–21, Figure 3). Direct stenting was performed in 92 (26%) patients. The primary end-point of in-stent minimal lumen diameter (MLD) at 8-month angiographic follow-up was significantly greater in the SES group (2.22 vs. 1.33 mm, $p<0.0001$), corresponding to a reduction in late lumen loss of 81% (0.2 vs. 1.05 mm, $p<0.0001$). This translated into a significantly reduced rate of restenosis, by 86% within the lesion (5.9 vs. 42.3%) and by 91% within the stent (3.9 vs. 41.7%).

Subacute thromboses (SAT) occurred in two patients in SES group; no SAT occurred in the control group ($p=0.25$). At 9-month clinical follow-up, total major adverse cardiac event rates were lower in SES compared with BMS (8.0 vs. 22.6 %, $p=0.0002$), principally owing to a significantly lower incidence of TLR (4.0 vs. 20.9%, relative reduction of 81%, $p<0.0001$). Thus, the results of the E-SIRIUS study showed how the benefit of SES over standard stents is maintained in a more complex cohort of patients, with lesions at a higher risk of restenosis.

The encouraging results obtained in clinical trials were also confirmed by reports of preliminary experience in real-life settings.

The pattern of restenosis occurring after implantation of SES has been evaluated in unselected lesions.[14] A total of 368 patients were treated with 841 SES in 741 lesions (slide 22). Mean lesion length was 17.48 ± 12.19 mm, mean stent length was 27.59 ± 14.02 mm, and mean reference vessel diameter was 2.69 ± 0.53 mm. Twenty-four patients returned for angiographic follow-up, 21 because of signs or symptoms of ischemia or a positive stress test, 2 for scheduled follow-up, and 1 for planned procedure on another vessel, at an average 4.1 ± 2.0 months from index procedure. Eleven patients had angiographic restenosis in 14 stented segments. Regarding the angiographic pattern of restenosis in these patients: all the restenotic lesions were focal, averaging 5.62 ± 1.90 mm in length (range 2.54–8.44 mm), and six of them were multifocal. This confirms the findings of the SIRIUS[11] trial, in which restenosis in sirolimus-eluting stents was found to be mostly focal. However, in contrast with the reports of the SIRIUS[11] study where restenotic lesions were located at the stent margins or in gaps between stents, all lesions were in the body of the stent, with the exception of one patient with multifocal lesions, one of which also involved the distal margin of a stent.

Morphological characteristics of in-SES restenosis have been evaluated also in the 'Rapamycin Eluting Stents Evaluated At Rotterdam Cardiology Hospital' the (RESEARCH) registry (slide 23).[15] An angiographic follow-up was obtained in 121 patients on a clinical basis or was scheduled at 6 months if complex lesions (left main, bifurcations, small vessels, chronic total occlusions, long stented segments, acute myocardial infarction, and in-stent restenotic lesions) had been treated. Angiograpic restenosis occurred in only 19 patients and 20 lesions, 1 of which were in-stent and 6 in the proximal edge. In five of the six patients with proximal edge restenosis, there was post-procedural evidence of injury (angiographic or IVUS dissection). Twelve of the 14 in-stent restenotic lesions were focal, 4 of which occurred in segments with gaps between stents or at stent fracture sites.

The effectiveness of SES in patients with multivessel disease has been recently reported (slides 24–26).[16] A total of 155 consecutive patients with 511 unselected lesions were treated with 573 SES. Number of lesions treated per patient was 3.3 ± 1.3 with a mean stent length of 87.4 ± 45.2 mm. At the 6-month clinical follow-up 3 patients (2.7%) died (only 1 death was cardiac), 4 patients (3.6%) had MI, and 16 patients (14.3%) with 24 lesions (6.7%) had TLR. Target-vessel revascularization (TVR) was required in 18 patients (16.1%) due to TLR of lesions treated with SES or to disease progression (1.8% of patients). The cumulative MACE rate was 22.3%. Cox regression analysis revealed total stent length per patient as the most powerful independent predictor of MACE. Overall stent thrombosis occurred in 3 patients (1.9%).

Recently, results from the RESEARCH registry have been published. In this series, a strategy of unrestricted usage of SES ($n=450$) was compared with conventional approaches that used bare stents in the pre-SES era in *de novo* lesions. Patients in the SES group more frequently had multivessel disease, more type-C lesions, received more stents, and had more bifurcation stenting. Although both study groups differed in some baseline and procedural characteristics, which may somewhat limit an unbiased comparison between them, it is worth noting that most if not all differences would be traditionally expected to increase the incidence of late complications in the SES-treated patients. Nevertheless, the treatment effect of SES was significantly higher than bare stents, remaining virtually unaffected after adjustment for procedural characteristics.

At 1 year, the cumulative rate of major adverse cardiac events (death, myocardial infarction, or target-vessel revascularization) was 9.7% in the SES group vs. 14.8% in the pre-SES group (hazard ratio (HR), 0.62 (95% CI 0.44–0.89); $p<0.008$). The 1-year risk of clinically driven target-vessel revascularization in the SES group and in the pre-SES group was 3.7 vs. 10.9%, respectively (HR, 0.35 (95% CI 0.21–0.57); $p<0.001$). A sub-group of complex patients ($n=238$) such as acute myocardial infarction, in-stent restenosis, small vessel, left main stenosis, chronic total occlusion, long lesions and bifurcations was analysed.[17] Binary in-segment restenosis in this high-risk group of patients was diagnosed in 7.9% of lesions (6.3% in-stent, 0.9% at the proximal edge, 0.7% at the distal edge). In-stent restenosis (OR 4.16, 95% CI 1.63–11.01; $p<0.01$), ostial location (OR 4.84, 95% CI 1.81–12.07; $p<0.01$), diabetes (OR 2.63, 95% CI 1.14–6.31; $p=0.02$), total stented length (per 10-mm increase; OR 1.42, 95% CI 1.21–1.68; $p<0.01$), reference diameter (per 1.0-mm increase; OR 0.46, 95% CI 0.24–0.87; $p=0.03$), and left anterior descending artery (OR 0.30, 95% CI 0.10–0.69; $p<0.01$) were identified as independent multivariate predictors.

In the registry of compassionate use of SES (the SECURE) registry[18] 250 patients with native or by-pass graft restenotic lesions received SES (slides 27–28). Primary end-point was TVF at 6 months. Fifty-two patients with prior radiation therapy failure (radiation) and 11 with no prior radiation therapy (no radiation) achieved 6 months follow-up. In the radiation group, 1.9% died, 5.8% had MI, and 20.5% had TLR with a TVF rate of 23.1%. On the other hand, in the no-radiation group, TLR was 8.8%, no patient died nor had MI, and TVF was 9%.

Arterial Revascularization Therapies Study part II (ARTS II) is a multicenter, European, open-label, non-randomized, stratified trial in about 45–50 centers which will include 600 eligible patients with multivessel disease who should be equally treatable by surgery or stenting with SES (slides 29–32). The results of ARTS II will be compared with the by-pass arm of Arterial Revascularization Therapies Study (ARTS I) as an historical control. A total of 606 patients were included in the study, mean stent/patients was 3.6, and inhibitors of IIb/IIIa glycoproteins were used only in 14.5% of the procedures. There were four acute thromboses and one subacute thrombosis.

'A Prospective, randomized, multi-center comparison of the Cypher Sirolimus-eluting and the Taxus paclitaxel-eluting stent systems' (the REALITY) trial has been recently completed. The REALITY trial compared the Taxus SR stent (Boston Scientific) with the Cypher stent (Cordis) in high-risk lesions. The primary end-point of this trial was binary angiographic in-lesion restenosis at 8 months, with more than 1300 patients enrolled in the trial. The sample size calculation assumed an angiographic in-lesion restenosis at 8 months of 14% for the Taxus vs. 8% for the Cypher.

The 'Future Revascularization Evaluation in patients Diabetes Mellitus Optimal management of Multivessel disease' (FREEDOM) trial will be evaluating SES implantation vs. CABG in diabetic patients with multivessel disease (slide 32). Primary end-point is 5-year mortality and MACE.

CONCLUSIONS

Drug-eluting stents have been demonstrated to decrease dramatically the rate of restenosis in randomized trials. Since April 2002, SES were marketed in Europe (since April 2003 in the USA), and paclitaxel-eluting stents received CE (Conformité Européenne) marking for commercialization in Europe in March 2003. However, at the present time, cost constraints and a lack of incremental reimbursement have limited their utilization in daily practice in many countries. Initial analyses of the SES, however, have shown a highly favorable cost-effectiveness profile in reducing repeat revascularization and combined major cardiac events, and encouraging results are coming from preliminary data from 'real-world use' of drug-eluting stents. A more comprehensive understanding of the impact of this new treatment in a wide variety of patients, as well as market competition with changes in the cost of these devices, is likely to redefine the relationship between costs and benefits.

REFERENCES

1. Serruys PW, de Jaegere P, Kiemeneij F, et al. A comparison of balloon-expandable-stent implantation with balloon angioplasty in patients with coronary artery disease. Benestent Study Group. N Engl J Med 1994; 331: 489–95
2. Fischman DL, Leon MB, Baim DS, et al. A randomized comparison of coronary-stent placement and balloon angioplasty in the treatment of coronary artery disease. Stent Restenosis Study Investigators. N Engl J Med 1994; 331: 496–501
3. Marx SO, Marks AR. Bench to bedside: the development of rapamycin and its application to stent restenosis. Circulation 2001; 104: 852–5
4. Serruys PW, Regar E, Carter AJ. Rapamycin eluting stent: the onset of a new era in interventional cardiology. Heart 2002; 87: 305–7
5. Sousa JE, Costa MA, Abizaid AC, et al. Sustained suppression of neointimal proliferation by sirolimus-eluting stents: one-year angiographic and intravascular ultrasound follow-up. Circulation 2001; 104: 2007–11
6. Degertekin M, Serruys PW, Foley DP, et al. Persistent inhibition of neointimal hyperplasia after sirolimus-eluting stent implantation: long-term (up to 2 years) clinical, angiographic, and intravascular ultrasound follow-up. Circulation 2002; 106: 1610–3
7. Sousa JE, Costa MA, Sousa AG, et al. Two-year angiographic and intravascular ultrasound follow-up after implantation of sirolimus-eluting stents in human coronary arteries. Circulation 2003; 107: 381–3

8. Regar E, Serruys PW, Bode C, et al. Angiographic findings of the multicenter Random-ized Study with the Sirolimus-Eluting Bx Velocity Balloon-Expandable Stent (RAVEL): sirolimus-eluting stents inhibit restenosis irrespective of the vessel size. Circulation 2002; 106: 1949–56

9. Morice MC, Serruys PW, Sousa JE, et al. A randomized comparison of a sirolimus-eluting stent with a standard stent for coronary revascularization. N Engl J Med 2002; 346: 1773–80

10. Abizaid A, Costa MA, Blanchard D, et al. Sirolimus-eluting stents inhibit neointimal hyperplasia in diabetic patients. Insights from the RAVEL Trial. Eur Heart J 2004; 25: 107–12

11. Moses JW, Leon MB, Popma JJ, et al. Sirolimus-eluting stents versus standard stents in patients with stenosis in a native coronary artery. N Engl J Med 2003; 349: 1315–23

12. Schofer J, Schluter M, Gershlick AH, et al. Sirolimus-eluting stents for treatment of patients with long atherosclerotic lesions in small coronary arteries: double-blind, randomized controlled trial (E-SIRIUS). Lancet 2003; 362: 1093–9

13. Holmes DR, Jr, Leon MB, Moses JW, et al. Analysis of 1-year clinical outcomes in the SIRIUS trial: a randomized trial of a sirolimus-eluting stent versus a standard stent in patients at high risk for coronary restenosis. Circulation 2004; 109: 634–40

14. Colombo A, Orlic D, Stankovic G, et al. Preliminary observations regarding angiographic pattern of restenosis after rapamycin-eluting stent implantation. Circulation 2003; 107: 2178–80

15. Lemos PA, Saia F, Ligthart JM, et al. Coronary restenosis after sirolimus-eluting stent implantation: morphological description and mechanistic analysis from a consecutive series of cases. Circulation 2003; 108: 257–60

16. Orlic D, Bonizzoni E, Stankovic G, et al. Treatment of multivessel coronary artery disease with sirolimus-eluting stent implantation: immediate and mid-term results. J Am Coll Cardiol 2004; 43: 1154–60

17. Lemos PA, Hoye A, Goedhart D, et al. Clinical, angiographic, and procedural predictors of angiographic restenosis after sirolimus-eluting stent implantation in complex patients: an evaluation from the Rapamycin-Eluting Stent Evaluated At Rotterdam Cardiology Hospital (RESEARCH) study. Circulation 2004; 109: 1366–70

18. Teirstein P. Cypher Compassionate Use – the SECURE Registry. Presented at the Scientific Sessions of the American College of Cardiology, Drug-Eluting Stent Symposium, Chicago, March 29, 2003

Taxus tips & tricks

Keith D Dawkins MD

The Taxus Program refers to a series of trials assessing the application of paclitaxel in the inhibition of in-stent restenosis in coronary artery lesions of increasing complexity (slide 1).

The Taxus technology consists of three integrated components: paclitaxel, a drug known to be effective in the inhibition of cellular proliferation; the Translute polymer offers controlled and predictable drug release; and the stent delivery platform, currently the Express^2 stent (slide 2).

Paclitaxel has a number of complex actions at the cellular level, principally affecting the microtubular dynamics involved in cell division. As a result, extracellular matrix synthesis and secretion is reduced, and smooth muscle cell proliferation and migration is attenuated, thus reducing the neointimal hyperplasia that results in in-stent restenosis (slide 3).

The paclitaxel effects on the cell cycle are dose-dependent. At the high doses used in oncology, cell death (apoptosis) may occur, but at the low doses applied to intra-coronary stents in the Taxus program, the primary effect is cytostatic. The typical paclitaxel dose used in the treatment of a patient with ovarian cancer is 3280 µg/kg, compared with 1.22 µg/kg in a patient treated with a 16 mm Taxus stent (slide 4).

Importantly, the dose of paclitaxel selected for the Taxus Program allows complete endothelial coverage of the stent struts, thus reducing the likelihood of late stent thrombosis (slide 5).

Scanning electron micrographs confirm the uniform endothelium with minimal platelet and leukocyte adhesion (slide 6).

The Translute polymer allows manipulation of the release kinetics of the paclitaxel. An early burst phase lasting 2 days is followed by a period of sustained low level release. By altering the polymer, the amount and pattern of paclitaxel release can be modified (slide 7).

Two formulations have been assessed: the slow release (SR) formulation is commercially available in Europe and the US and has been studied in Taxus I, II, III, IV and V. The moderate release (MR) formulation, which is currently under investigation, delivers a three times higher local drug dose and was used in Taxus VI, and was compared with the SR formulation in Taxus II (slide 8).

The two different release formulations have been applied to a variety of lesion subsets, from short discrete lesions treated with a single stent, to long complex disease treated with multiple overlapping stents. The early Taxus trials used a new intravascular rigid (NIR) stent mounted on a Conformer balloon, whereas the more recent trials use the Express[2] stent platform (slide 9).

The application of a carrier matrix allows for programmable release kinetics, together with uniform, durable and predictable drug distribution, in comparison with systems that apply the drug coating directly to the stent (slide 10).

The carrier itself provides challenges in the manufacturing process in relation to mechanical integrity and vascular compatibility. It is important that the carrier itself does not provoke a foreign body reaction (slide 11).

Taxus I (slide 12).

Following detailed animal model assessment, Taxus I was the first human evaluation of a polymer-based paclitaxel eluting intracoronary stent (slide 13).

Taxus I was a safety and efficacy trial using the slow release (SR) formulation of paclitaxel loaded on a NIRx stent mounted on a Conformer balloon randomized 1:1 to treatment with an uncoated NIR stent. The primary endpoint was 30 day MACE which was 0%, with a 6-month binary restenosis rate of 0% in the NIRx group compared with 10% in the NIR group (slide 14).

Six-month QCA favored the NIRx with a significantly larger MLD and lower diameter stenosis (slide 15, Figure 1).

Late loss was 0.71 mm in the control NIR stent group and 0.35 mm in the NIRx group (slide 16).

The Taxus I trial confirmed the safety and efficacy of the paclitaxel-eluting NIRx stent in the treatment of short, discrete *de novo* lesions (slide 17).

Taxus II (slide 18).

Taxus II compared the safety and efficacy of two consecutive cohorts of patients treated with the slow release (SR) and moderate release (MR) NIRx stent in the treatment in lesions < 12 mm in length in vessels 3.0–3.5 mm in diameter (slide 19).

The primary endpoint of Taxus II was percent in-stent net volume obstruction assessed by IVUS. The primary endpoint was reached with a 60% relative reduction, similar in the SR and MR groups (slide 20, Figure 2).

The secondary endpoint was 6-month binary restenosis. There was a significant reduction in binary restenosis in patients treated with the NIRx stent without delete-rious edge effects. There was no significant difference in the effectiveness of the SR and MR preparation (slide 21).

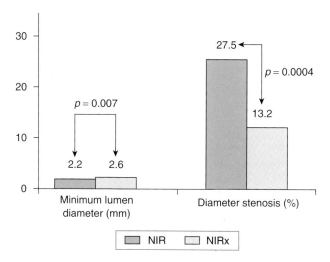

Figure 1   Taxus I: Angiographic results (6 months)

MACE-free survival improved over time with a delta of 8.8% at 6 months increasing to 10.5% at 12 months (slide 22, Figure 3).

The reduction in MACE was due to a sustained reduction in TLR, with no significant difference between the two preparations (slide 23).

Taxus III (slide 24).

Taxus III was a 30-patient registry undertaken in two centers in Germany assessing the feasibility of treating in-stent restenosis with a drug eluting paclitaxel stent (slide 25).

For this high-risk subgroup, 30 day MACE was low with no deaths and a non-Q wave infarct rate of 3.4% (slide 26).

Detailed 6-month assessment with Optical Coherence Tomography (OCT) demonstrated the typical 'stent-within-a-stent' appearance, and the neointima formation within the drug-eluting stent can be clearly seen, thus reducing the likelihood of late stent thrombosis from exposed stent struts (slide 27).

Taxus IV (slide 28).

In the Taxus IV trial, 1326 patients were randomized 1:1 between treatment with a Taxus Express stent and an untreated Express (control) stent. Lesion length by visual estimate was 10–28 mm, in vessels with a reference diameter of 2.5–3.75 mm (slide 29).

TLR fell significantly in the Taxus treated patients at 9 months angiographic follow-up (slide 30, Figure 4).

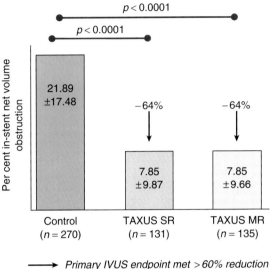

Figure 2   Taxus II: 6-month IVUS endpoint

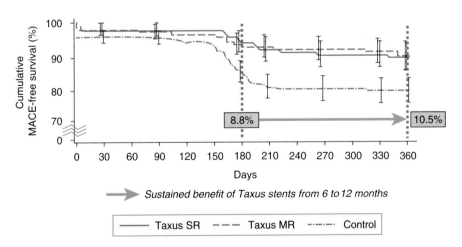

Figure 3   Taxus II: 12-month MACE-free survival

There was a significant increase in the TLR rate in the control group between 9 and 12 months with a delta of 9.3% increasing to 10.7% (slide 31, Figure 5).

In the Taxus group, TLR was independent of lesion length or reference vessel diameter (slide 32).

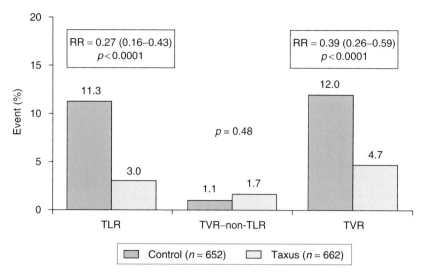

Figure 4 Taxus IV: TLR and TVR (9 months)

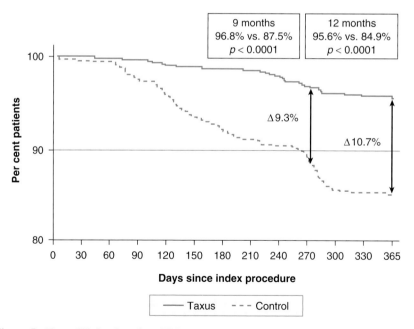

Figure 5 Taxus IV: freedom from TLR

The favorable impact of the Taxus stent on TLR in Taxus IV was uniform across all lesion and patient subgroups (slide 33).

Taxus V (slide 34).

The Taxus V trial is the US randomized pivotal expansion trial which addresses the applicability of the Taxus Express^2 SR stent in the treatment of long lesions and small vessels. Recruitment is complete and the results will be presented in late 2354 (slide 35).

Despite the favorable results in Taxus III, the efficacy of drug elution vis-à-vis intravascular brachytherapy for the treatment of in-stent restenosis remains unclear. Taxus V ISR is a randomized trial comparing the Taxus Express^2 SR stent with intravascular brachytherapy using a beta source. The primary endpoint is 9 months TVR. Recruitment is on going (slide 36).

Taxus VI (slide 37).

Taxus II demonstrated comparable safety and efficacy of the slow and moderate release formulations of paclitaxel, but the outcomes in more complex disease were unknown. Taxus VI addressed this issue using the MR preparation (slide 38).

The mean lesion length in the Taxus VI trial was 20.6 mm, with a total stent length of 33.4 mm. More than half the patients had complex (ACC Type C) disease, small vessel disease accounted for more than a quarter, overlapping stents were used in more than a quarter, and multivessel disease was treated in 23.5% of patients. A fifth of the patients were diabetic (slide 39).

Patients were randomized 1:1 between a Taxus Express^2 MR stent and an uncoated Express^2 control stent. Nine-month clinical follow-up was 98% complete (slide 40).

Patient demographics were well matched in the two groups. One and a half stents were used per patient, and the stent/lesion length ratio was long at 1.8 in the control group and 1.7 in the Taxus MR group (slide 41).

The primary endpoint of the study was met with a 53% reduction in TVR at 9 months reduced from 19.4 to 9.1% (slide 42, Figure 6).

Actuarial event free survival demonstrates the increasing TLR benefit over time with a delta of 12.4% at 9 months (slide 43, Figure 7).

MACE composition at nine months was similar in the two groups which would be anticipated in this long complex lesion trial (slide 44).

The Taxus MR stent was effective over the range of classic risk factors which are known to be associated with an adverse TLR rate (slide 45).

Potential concerns over stent thrombosis was not realized in the Taxus VI trial. Importantly, no stent thromboses were demonstrated in the 3-month period following cessation of treatment with clopidogrel (slide 46).

Nine-month QCA analysis was assessed using standard techniques and was described independently for the stented segment and the analysis segment (i.e. the stented segment plus 5 mm at either end) (slide 47).

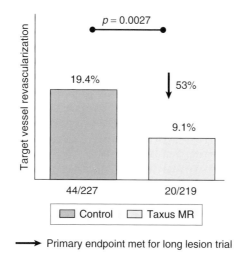

Figure 6 Taxus VI: TVR at 9 months

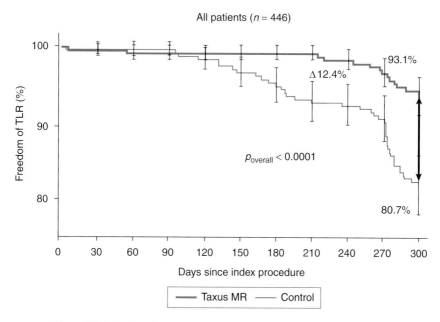

Figure 7 Taxus VI: TLR benefit over time

The diameter stenosis benefit with the Taxus MR stent was seen both in the stented segment and at the edges (slide 48).

Consistency of in-stent late loss at 0.39 mm has been seen across the Taxus trials and was not adversely affected by the long complex lesions treated in Taxus VI (slide 49).

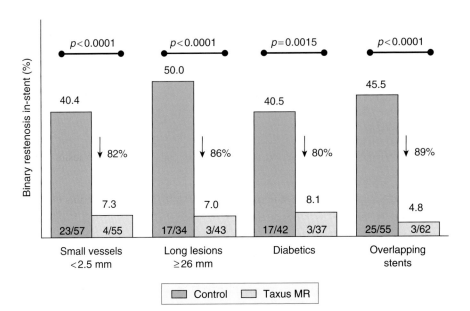

Figure 8   Taxus VI: restenosis benefit independent of classic risk factors

The distribution of late loss demonstrated the characteristic left shift in the Taxus MR treated group with little evidence of positive remodeling (i.e. negative late loss) (slide 50).

An impressive 72% relative reduction in binary restenosis from 32.9 to 9.1% was noted at 9 months (slide 51).

The improvement in binary restenosis was evident in the stented segment with no deleterious effects at the edges (slide 52).

Binary restenosis was independent of classic risk factors (slide 53, Figure 8).

The binary restenosis rate in the Express[2] (control) arm of Taxus VI is in accord with the other long lesion trials using bare metal stents (slide 54).

In the 19 patients that did experience in-stent restenosis in the Taxus MR group, the length of the ISR was significantly shorter than in the 63 patients with ISR in the control group (slide 55).

Furthermore, the pattern of restenosis in the Taxus MR group was more focal, favoring repeat conventional treatment with percutaneous intervention (slide 56).

Late aneurysm formation as a manifestation of positive remodeling is a potential concern with drug-eluting stents. There was no significant difference in the incidence of late acquired aneurysm formation between the Taxus MR and control groups at 9 months, despite using a very conservative definition of aneurysm of only 1.2 times reference vessel diameter (slide 57).

Lesion length is a recognized cause of an increase in TLR rate in patients treated with plain metallic stents. This was reflected in the control arm of the Taxus VI trial. However, there was a fall in TLR rate with increasing lesion length in the patients treated with the Taxus MR stent (slide 58).

This was reflected in the reduction in binary restenosis in relation to lesion length (slide 59).

Overall, 2289 patients have been recruited in the Taxus II, IV and VI trials of whom 458 (20%) have been diabetic (slide 60).

This powerful diabetic dataset demonstrates the consistent benefit of the Taxus stent on TLR in diabetics including those treated with insulin (slide 61).

In patients treated with the Taxus stent, binary restenosis in diabetics at 5.1% is not significantly different to non-diabetics at 4.9% (slide 62).

In the era of plain metallic stents, the concept of 'spot stenting' was advocated because of the known relationship between stent length and the likelihood of restenosis. With the advent of drug elution, operators favor 'stenting long' (i.e. from angiographically 'normal' vessel on either side of the lesion) to avoid geographic miss. It is apparent from the Taxus VI trial that there may be an optimal stent/lesion ratio of 1.6–1.9 (slide 63).

Future directions of the Taxus Program will include the assessment of the new Liberté stent platform in the ATLAS trial, the application of the Taxus MR stent in primary intervention in acute myocardial infarction in the HORIZON trial, and the treatment of multivessel disease (including left main stem) in the SYNTAX trial (slide 64).

The Liberté stent combines many of the features of the Express[2] stent on thinner stainless steel struts with continuous cell architecture on three platforms (slide 65).

The ATLAS trial will assess a wide range of lesions treated with the Liberté stent, comparing the TLR outcome with a historical control from Taxus IV and V (slide 66).

HORIZON will be the first trial in which the Taxus stent is used in the primary treatment of acute myocardial infarction. A sub-study will assess the optimal anti-thrombotic regimen comparing unfractionated heparin plus a IIb/IIIa inhibitor to bivalirudin and bail out IIb/IIIa inhibitor (slide 67).

The SYNTAX trial has a novel design in which consecutive patients with three-vessel disease including left main lesions will be randomized between PCI and surgical revascularization; patients deemed unsuitable for randomization will be followed in either the PCI or CABG registry **(slide 68)**.

SYNTAX will provide the evidence base for or against surgical conversion to PCI **(slide 69)**.

The planned Taxus trials will address the difficult lesion subsets which are becoming more common as interventional cardiologists treat more 'surgical' disease **(slide 70)**.

2

General Approach with Drug-Eluting Stents

Antonio Colombo MD

INTRODUCTION

The most important step when implanting a drug-eluting stent is to be able to get the stent to the lesion. Stenting with DES is not only performed to improve the immediate result or to cover a dissection, it is mainly performed in order to avoid restenosis. This means that the stent is a therapeutic option in percutaneous coronary intervention (PCI), and each lesion dilated needs to be stented (slide 2).

A second aspect is to select the appropriate length of the stent and, I would add, the appropriate size. The goal is to make the procedure safe, basically to avoid any risk of thrombosis by paying attention to appropriate antiplatelet therapy and optimal stent implantation, and finally to make it effective by avoiding restenosis.

In order to get the stent to the lesion, it is important to select the appropriate guiding catheter, not to be afraid to predilate sometimes fairly aggressively and, in some situations, to consider rotational atherectomy and, finally, to utilize a second wire (buddy-wire). When we utilize a second wire, we always deliver the stent on the softer wire and leave the support wire like 'iron-man' or 'stabilizer' as a buddy-wire (slide 3).

It may be possible that, in the future, with the advent of more flexible and lower-profile drug-eluting stents, some of the delivery problems will be improved. However, they will never be completely solved, because a stent will always be more rigid and difficult to deliver compared with a balloon (slide 4).

The importance of full lesion coverage and selecting the appropriate stent lengths is highlighted when we compare the 'old' US-SIRIUS to the 'new' Canadian and European SIRIUS. It is clear that there is an improvement in the restenosis rate, even if it is not statistically significant in the group treated with the sirolimus stent. This improvement occurred despite the fact that the lesions in the 'new' SIRIUS were located in the vessels with the small reference size (slide 5).

One major reason for this better performance is illustrated in slide 5, where we see that the proximal margin binary restenosis and the distal margin binary restenosis rates are better, with significant p value for the proximal margin. The use of long stents is most probably an explanation for this finding (slide 6).

What about direct stenting? Our views on this method are in favor of direct stenting in all situations in which it can be applied safely. The DIRECT trial demonstrates that the performance of direct stenting, as regards 8-month late loss and composite events, is not at all inferior, and may be even slightly superior, to standard stenting with pre-dilatation. This, of course, applies to lesions suitable for this approach (slide 7).

Slide 8 demonstrates that the binary restenosis with direct stenting was similar and may be slightly better, particularly for the in-lesion binary restenosis compared with standard stent.

Slide 9 demonstrates that the clinical events at 6 months were similar at less than 5% with either direct or standard stenting.

SIMPLE LESIONS

For simple lesions, our approach is to make it simple. This will be demonstrated in the few cases we present as simple lesion treatment, which highlight the value of direct stenting when possible or the value of gentle pre-dilatation.

Slides 11–14 show a lesion in which gentle pre-dilatation was performed with the final result following stenting shown.

Slides 15–18 show another lesion in which stent length was evaluated following a gentle pre-dilatation which prompted for usage of a longer stent.

Slides 19–22 show a further example of a lesion treated with simple pre-dilatation and then stenting.

Pre-dilatation approach

We must state that no final word is out regarding the best approach to pre-dilate a lesion: gentle pre-dilatation, full pre-dilatation, use of cutting balloon, or use of the Fx Minirail balloon (Guidant). Our impression is that in complex lesions, a more aggressive pre-dilatation approach should be used, while in simple lesions, a more conservative and simple approach could be of advantage. We should never forget the usage of rotational atherectomy in very calcified lesions. If the 1.5-mm balloon does not cross, do not hesitate to consider rotablation.

COMPLEX LESIONS

Now, moving on to more complex lesions, the issue of lesion preparation becomes, in our view, the most important aspect.

Before entering into the technical aspects of the procedure, it is important to evaluate the duration of antiplatelet therapy as demonstrated in slide 24. We regard this slide with great respect, because, particularly, when dealing with a complex lesion, it is of the utmost importance to be sure that the patient will be able to tolerate double antiplatelet therapy for an extended period of time.

We set different time lengths: 3 months for single or multiple Cypher stents up to 33 mm, and longer periods of time for more complex lesions or for left main or for usage of Taxus stents.

Bifurcational lesions

The first set of lesions we would like to discuss is bifurcational lesions.

As shown in slide 26, the first consideration when dealing with a bifurcational lesion is to ask ourselves: are we going to use one stent or two?

The answer to this question comes by answering multiple questions and then making a balanced judgment according to how many of these questions were answered in a positive or negative fashion. Slide 26 shows a series of questions for which the answer will condition the operator more towards one stent versus/or two stents.

'How large and important is a side branch?' If the side branch is very important and large, we may condition for two stents. On the other hand, another question comes up: is the side branch diseased or not? If the side branch is large and diseased, we would certainly go for two stents. If the side branch is only large, but not diseased, we may stay with one stent.

Answering each of those questions gives a general idea, but we are far from making a score, and the decision is almost always a decision that the operator takes based on his own experience. As the slides point out, sometimes a decision should be made only following pre-dilatation of both the main branch and the side branch. It is important, as said in slide 27, to re-evaluate the need for two stents after pre-dilatation of both the main branch and the side branch.

Of course, we like to limit direct stenting to simple lesions, and we are far from advocating this approach in bifurcational lesions. The step to dilate the side branch is dependent on the amount of disease present at the ostium of the side branch. As slide 28 points out, when we decide to treat both branches of the bifurcation, they should be treated with drug-eluting stents utilizing one of the two approaches, crush or V-technique. We have now completely abandoned the T-stenting technique or the culotte technique, and when two stents are implanted, we utilize one of the two above techniques.

Slide 29 shows a typical lesion for which we would consider two stents. There is a severe narrowing in the obtuse marginal branch and almost an occlusion in the distal circumflex. We feel that this lesion would not respond very well to a single stent. The same considerations apply to the lesion presented in slide 30: the diagonal is very large, has a disease distal to the situation, which can be covered by a long stent, and both branches, left anterior descending (LAD) and diagonal, are severely diseased in the proximal part. Slide 31 shows the result following the crush technique and kissing inflation. Slide 32 shows another example of lesion in which we advocate usage of more than one stent; a distal left main with an intermediate branch and circumflex. We propose the treatment in this case could be the crush technique or V-technique with three arms. Slides 33 and 34 show deployment of three stents with the crush approach utilizing a 9-Fr guide-catheter. The last stent to be inflated, as shown in slide 34, is always at the more proximal stent; in this case, the LAD stent. Slides 35–37 show the final result and the 6-month follow up.

In slide 38, we demonstrate a reverse crush, which is an approach utilized for provisional stenting of the side branch. In this case, the stenosis at the ostium of the left anterior descending demonstrated in slide 39 was treated with a single stent going from the left main to the LAD (slide 40). The result is shown in slide 37. The ostium of the large intermediate branch is suboptimal. Despite balloon dilatation of this branch as shown in slide 41, the result did not improve; as a matter of fact there is a slight dissection, as shown in slide 42. At this point, we decided to perform reverse crush by advancing a stent into the side branch, and crush in the protruding part of the stent with a bare balloon, positioned in the main branch (slides 43, 44). The crush of the protruding stent is demonstrated in slide 45. The result is shown in slide 46. This procedure should always be completed with re-dilatation of the side branch and kissing (slide 43). The final result is shown in slides 48 and 49.

Various types of crush technique are summarized in slide 50. The main technical consideration when performing the crush technique is to be very meticulous to always perform final kissing; in our experience, final kissing is required in almost 100% of cases at the present time (slide 51).

More important or equally as important as final kissing, is also to perform final high-pressure dilatation in the side branch before final kissing. The section of this book by Dr John Ormiston highlights the importance of the added maneuver to improve the result of the crush technique. Slide 52 shows how many struts impede the ostium of the side branch if kissing is not performed. The struts that can be seen through the dilated struts in the second frame are located on the opposite wall of the main branch. Final kissing not only improves the position of the struts, but also improves the lumen gain. Slide 53 shows the large lumen gain obtained in the main branch and in the side branch following final kissing, abbreviated in this slide as FK. This benefit will translate into a lower restenosis rate. Our current experience in patients treated with final kissing and the crush technique is summarized in slide 54, where we detected 15% focal restenosis with only 7% target lesion revascularization. Slides 55–64 show an example of treatment of multiple bifurcations with a crush technique, with a very gratifying follow up at 8 months.

What is important to reinforce is the fact that many times, even if we see angiographic restenosis at the ostium of the side branch, this restenosis is very focal and is clinically not relevant. Slide 65 demonstrates that, despite angiographic restenosis at the ostium, the diagonal branch pressure wire measurement following adenosine administration did not show any abnormal fractional flow reserve, which maintained the value of 0.91.

As mentioned previously, the V-technique is another option for the treatment of bifurcations. Slides 66–74 demonstrate two cases in which the V-technique was used. A V-technique is very simple and is very easily performed. The decision as to when to use the V-technique or the crush approach is discussed in slide 75. We would use the V-technique in a very proximal lesion with minimal disease proximal to the side where the V is performed, and it may be problematic and sometimes difficult to place a stent proximally to a lesion stented with a V-technique. The most common approach to deal with this problem is to convert the V of the side branch into a crush and then post-dilate with kissing in the side branch.

Left main lesions

We have treated this type of lesion with drug-eluting stents in 43 patients (slide 77). Many of these patients had lesions located at the distal bifurcation. It is also worth mentioning that a number of these patients presented with left main restenosis following placement of bare-metal stents. Our initial findings are summarized in slide 78, where the in-hospital MACE is very low owing to the ease of delivery of these stents. The 6-month MACE (slide 79) is acceptable but is affected by two problems: (1) the fact that the stent thrombosis occurs when the patient has to stop double antiplatelet therapy before the stated time (one event was due to this complication), and (2) the fact that the rate of restenosis, despite being low, is still in double digits (23% in our experience). It is worth mentioning that restenosis, although focal and relatively benign, still demands a second intervention. Slide 80 summarizes all our cases of restenosis. It is interesting to note that in many cases, the lesion involved a bifurcation, and diabetes was frequently present.

Another unique element is the fact that in a few cases, only one 3.5-mm Cypher stent was used. Slide 81 shows that diabetes was one of the major offenders; five out of the six patients with diabetes required a revascularization. Slides 82–98 present various cases of restenosis following stenting of the left main. The final case illustrates a thrombotic event occurring at 5 months following discontinuation of double antiplatelet therapy, originally prescribed for 3 months. Despite being rare, we cannot dismiss the fact that this complication occasionally may occur. The most interesting finding in our cases of restenosis is the fact that the restenotic events do not always occur at the site where the lesion is or was more severe, and even in bifurcations the restenotic lesion sometimes occurs distal to the bifurcation or in a straight segment.

Multivessel disease

Treatment of multivessel disease brings into the equation the fact that many lesions are treated in a single patient. This brings into play the cumulative risk of restenosis which, even if low per lesion, increases when we calculate per patient. Slides 100–102 show treatment of a patient in various segments of different vessels with multiple Cypher stents. It is pleasing to note that at 10 months, no restenosis is present in any treated vessel.

Our experience in multivessel disease has been summarized in recent publication by Dr Orlic.[1] The important element of this study is the fact that the target-vessel revascularization per patient was 16% at 6 months, highlighting the fact that multiple lesions are present in the single patient with a target-lesion revascularization per lesion which was low (6.7%), but unfortunately additive (slide 103).

The plus side concerning restenosis in drug-eluting stents is summarized in slide 104, which shows that the restenotic event is almost always very focal when occurring inside the stent. In this slide, the number on top of the blue dots represents the length of the restenotic event. There are various theories or hypotheses as to why restenosis can occur. Slide 105 presents a diagram which serves to highlight the fact that proliferation may perhaps occur in the areas devoid of drugs, where the stent struts are not homogeneously distributed and a drug delivery may not occur. Slide 106 shows a complex lesion treated with multiple stents. The follow-up results at 9 months show a restenosis at different sites. As demonstrated in slide 107, we had the opportunity to evaluate these multiple restenosis by intravascular ultrasound, and the findings are demonstrated in slides 108–111. In all these slides, we see various possible causes: a gap in slide 108, a stent underexpansion in slide 109, struts maldistribution in slide 110, and a severe maldistribution in slide 111.

One important element to bare in mind is shown in slide 112: in this case, we demonstrate that even post-dilatation cannot correct a strut maldistribution. The increase in the lumen cross-sectional area may occur without improving the symmetry of the stent and the strut distribution. Slide 113 demonstrates the association between restenosis and the events called no-struts. Despite the use of a long stent, IVUS fails to demonstrate any strut at the site of restenosis. It is very possible, as reported in the literature, that strut rupture could be an explanation for these phenomena.

The current working hypothesis is summarized in slide 114, in which gap, asymmetric strut distribution (through excessive distance of struts through the target area; media or adventitia) and, in addition, strut rupture may be possible causes of restenosis. As demonstrated in slide 115, stent over-dilatation may not necessarily improve strut distribution and sometimes may even cause a deterioration. One final element that we want to bring attention to is polymer rupture (slide 116), which, even if not clearly emphasized, may contribute to this focal restenosis.

Slides 117 and 118 demonstrate how the cells of the two current drug-eluting stents, Taxus Express (Boston Scientific) and Bx Velocity (Cordis), are highly dependent on the final diameter that the stent achieves. It is also reasonably intuitive regarding the possibility that, inside the cell areas, drug under-dosing may occur owing to uneven distribution of the cell strut, particularly in calcific fibrotic lesions or in areas with a severe angulation. The suggestions that we would like to make to conclude this discussion are presented below. However, our conclusions are still in evolution, and we would like to stress the fact that further experience and trials may change these suggestions.

Suggestions (in evolution)

- Stent from normal-to-normal (near-normal)
  - This will lower or eliminate peri-stent restenosis
- You are utilizing long stents and much metal: be aware of thrombosis
  - Do not under-deploy
  - Do not leave residual dissections
  - *If in doubt, post-dilate*, but always stay in the stent margins
  - Evaluate correct clopidogrel pretreatment
- In-stent restenosis: a new entity without a clear explanation
  - Avoid gaps (mis-labelled in-stent restenosis)
  - Try to obtain symmetric stent expansion
  - Stent homogeneous distribution
  - Stent contact to vessel wall
  - Optimal stent expansion
  - Prepare the lesion in selected cases
  - IVUS guidance and documentary studies are needed
- Direct stenting versus pre-dilatation
  - Remember that no advantages of direct stenting versus pre-dilatation (besides cost and time) have been demonstrated
  - If possible, perform direct stenting
  - If in doubt: pre-dilate
  - In complex lesions: pre-dilate
- How should we pre-dilate?
  - Focal pre-dilation: yes
  - Complete pre-dilatation or just to allow delivery?
  - Do not forget that RTB is ideal for preparation of very calcified lesions: *the easiest way to deliver a stent is to have the lesion well prepared*

REFERENCE

1. Orlic D, Bonizzoni E, Stankovic G, et al. Treatment of multivessel coronary artery disease with sirolimus-eluting stent implantation: immediate and mid-term results. J Am Coll Cardiol 2004; 43: 1154–60

3

Lesion-Specific Stenting

SIMPLE LESIONS

DIRECT STENTING IS ENCOURAGED

When dealing with focal lesions, we have to take all the advantages presented by the simplicity of the situation. This means that when the lesion is described as non-calcified and, particularly in the context of single- or double-vessel disease, a consideration for direct stenting should be strongly made. The general principle about direct stenting should not be forgotten, which is 'if in doubt, don't do it'. If the operator feels comfortable and believes that the lesion can be stented directly, this should be done without fear of increasing acute or long-term complications or deteriorating the results.

The first case that we demonstrate (**# 11844**) shows a lesion in the mid of the left anterior descending, which is suitable for direct stenting, because it is not particularly tortuous and neither does it appear calcified (slide 1 (*frames 1–3*)). A stent 3.5 mm in diameter, 18 mm long (Cypher stent, Cordis) is deployed with an excellent final result.

The same situation is shown in a second case (**# 11677**; slide 2 (*frames 1–4*)) with a variation due to the placement of a filter device because of the unstable clinical symptoms of this patient, suggesting a possible complex and thrombotic lesion. This is an additional element to perform during direct stenting. The right coronary artery in *frame 1* shows the described lesion, which is effectively treated with a single 3.5-mm Taxus stent (Boston Scientific).

The concept of direct stenting has been supported by a recently completed trial, the DIRECT study, which is a multi-center prospective nonrandomized trial evaluating the feasibility of direct stenting and comparing the results with historical controls from the SIRIUS Cypher study (slides 3–5). The primary end-point of this study was the 8-month QCA late loss and the 30-day events. As shown in slides 3–5, the direct group performs very well with a 0.21 mm late loss by QCA at 8 months, which was not different from the control group (0.24 mm). In addition, in terms of the 30-day event and angina, there was no difference.

Regarding 8-months binary restenosis, single digits were applicable to both the stent and the lesion, with a slight numerical advantage for direct stenting, with 6% binary restenosis in-lesion analysis. Overall, we can safely state that direct stenting can be performed when technically feasible.

MINIMIZATION OF TRAUMA

When the lesion is reasonably severe and the operator does not feel comfortable with direct stenting, then comes pre-dilatation. This is still a big debate: should we perform gentle pre-dilatation or full, aggressive pre-dilatation?

We present a case of gentle pre-dilatation (**Case # 10813; slides 1–4** (*frames 1–8*)), but again we are not so sure that this approach is exactly the best. Unfortunately, only a prospective dedicated trial will be able to answer this question. The lesion in the circumflex presented in *frame 1* and *frame 2*, is reasonably severe and is not suitable for direct stenting. An approach of gentle pre-dilatation is taken: a 1.5-mm balloon is utilized as shown in *frame 4* and then a 33-mm-long Cypher stent is deployed as shown in *frame 6*. Notice that *frame 5* shows a modest pre-dilatation, which is what you can expect following the usage of a 1.5-mm balloon. The final result is presented in *frames 7* and *8*.

The second case chosen to illustrate the value and importance of pre-dilatation is a right coronary artery presented in *frames 1* and *2* (**Case # 11659; slides 5–8** (*frames 1–8*)), where a severe distal lesion is present. The lesion is pre-dilated with a 1.5-mm balloon with an acceptable immediate result presented in *frame 4*. Following pre-dilatation, a 33-mm-long Cypher stent is deployed and shown in *frames 5* and *6*. The final results are presented in *frames 7* and *8*.

At present, we have no data to support this conduct of operation except the intuition, based on our experience, that a gentle pre-dilatation may prevent excessive trauma. When dealing with a more calcified form of fibrotic lesion, this approach may not be suitable. Unfortunately, it is not always possible to know *a priori* if a lesion will respond well to gentle pre-dilatation or will require a more aggressive approach.

FULL LESION COVERAGE

Full lesion coverage is a newcomer, brought into the field by the use of drug-eluting stents. In the history of stenting, we moved from full lesion coverage, which was initially proposed, to a more selective lesion coverage in order to minimize stent length. With the emergence of drug-eluting stents, we reverted to the concept of stenting from healthy to healthy. It is not rare, when we examine the results of various trials, to notice a tremendous mismatch between stent length and lesion length. This is justified by the goal of minimizing the risk of peri-stent restenosis. The example of a discrete lesion of the circumflex treated with a 28-mm Taxus stent as shown in *frames 1* and *2* brings these concepts into light (**Case # 11632; slide 1** (*frames 1–3*)). The final result, presented in *frame 3*, shows an excellent peri-stent result that is neither step up nor step down. This concept is almost totally eliminated with the use of drug-eluting stents.

The next lesion, presented in *frames 1* and *2* of a right coronary artery, illustrates a strategic decision taken not as a baseline, but following pre-dilatation (**Case # 10825; slides 2–5** (*frames 1–8*)). This relatively discrete lesion of the right coronary artery was predilated with a 2.0-mm balloon and, following this step, the lesion appears to be longer, perhaps owing to some plaque shift or trauma created by the dilating balloon. This finding prompted usage of a long stent as shown in *frames 5* and *6*. The lesion was treated with a 3.5 × 32-mm Taxus stent, with a final result presented in *frames 7* and *8*. Two aspects are shown: (1) full lesion coverage, and (2) evaluation of the stent length not as a baseline, but following pre-dilatation when this procedure needs to be performed.

APPROPRIATE SIZING

When dealing with a simple lesion, we should not forget the value of appropriate stent sizing. Appropriate stent sizing is important, particularly when using the Cypher stent, because this stent changes in stent geometry when going from a 3-mm stent to a 3.5-mm stent (from six cells to seven cells).

The lesion presented in *frame 1* (**Case # 11708; slide 1** (*frames 1–4*)) is a discrete lesion of an intermediate branch, which was evaluated following pre-dilatation as shown in *frame 2*; it was decided to use a 3.5-mm stent rather than a 3-mm Cypher stent. The decision may be important, because better lesion coverage means also a more homogeneous delivery of the drug.

The same concept is illustrated in *frames 1* and *2* of a long left anterior descending (LAD) lesion (**Case # 11826; slides 2–4** (*frames 1–6*)). In this case, the stent utilized was the Taxus stent, for which the stent design is the same if we go from a 2.25-mm stent up to a 3.5-mm stent. This uniformity of cell number and stent design from 2.25 to 3.5 mm could bring into criticism the concept of optimizing stent size, because the value of better drug distribution may not always be supported if we are using the same stent. Nevertheless, utilizing a larger balloon could potentially always be advantageous, because the final lumen is larger and probably the final result superior. The long lesion in the left anterior descending presented in *frames 1* and *2* has been treated with a long Taxus stent 3.5 mm in diameter, with the final result presented in *frames 5* and *6*.

COMPLEX LESIONS
PART I – BIFURCATIONAL LESIONS

Introduction: practical approaches to bifurcational lesions

Antonio Colombo MD, *Goran Stankovic* MD, *Giovanni Martini* RT

The first question that needs to be addressed when stenting a bifurcation is whether one or two stents need to be used. We propose several aspects that the operator should consider in order to make a balanced judgment to help answer this main question. Here we list several considerations which should be evaluated in order to draw up a final plan:

- How large and important is the side branch?
- Does the side branch come out from the main at an acute angle?
- Does the ostium or the proximal segment of the side branch have a significant narrowing?
- Is the side branch very difficult to wire?
- Is the patient a very high-risk patient and does the side branch appear relatively important?
- Is the main branch severely narrowed with a considerable plaque burden?

If the answer is YES the operator will lean more towards two stents.
  Sometimes a decision should be made only following pre-dilatation of the main branch and of the side branch.
  Some important considerations should also be kept in mind:

- There is a limited role for direct stenting in bifurcational lesions
- Wire both branches before dilating the main branch (most of the time)
- Dilate the main branch to evaluate how the side branch behaves
- Dilate the side branch only if it is diseased or if it significantly deteriorates after dilatation of the main branch

Table 1 Treatment of the side branch: proposed treatment according to the specific conditions and size of the side branch

	Side branch		
Specific conditions	<2.0 mm	2–3 mm	>3.0 mm
Threatened side-branch occlusion	Wire protection or no protection	Wire protection Pre-dilate before stenting the main branch	Wire protection Pre-dilate and/or debulk Plan to stent both branches
Nonthreatened side branch	No wire protection	No wire protection	No wire protection
Side branch significantly compromised after main-branch balloon dilatation	Only if clinically indicated, wire and pre-dilate before stenting the main branch	Wire and pre-dilate If >2.5 mm, consider stenting both branches	Wire and pre-dilate Plan to stent both branches
Side branch significantly compromised after main-branch stenting	Only if clinically indicated, wire and dilate	Particularly if flow impaired or closed, try to wire and dilate If >2.5 mm, consider bailout stent for through struts	Stent both branches

During interventions in bifurcational lesions, any side branch of ≥2.0 mm should be preserved. Side branches of ≥2.0 mm in diameter with ostial disease or at risk for plaque shift should, in our opinion, be treated with elective balloon dilatation. The size of the side branch is determined operationally. This means that any side branch for which the operator may consider using a balloon of 2 mm or larger in diameter will need to be preserved. Side branches of smaller size (1.5-mm balloon) should be preserved only if clinically relevant. Table 1 illustrates the approach we use to protect the side branch in several anatomic settings.

We distinguish between elective side-branch treatment with balloon dilatation followed by conditional stenting and the bailout treatment of a side branch that was compromised following dilatation of the main branch. This may prevent side-branch occlusion following stent placement on the major branch and may facilitate rewiring the side branch through the struts of the stent. In our opinion, true bifurcation stenting with elective stent implantation of both the main and the side branch should be performed only in cases in which the side branch is ≥2.5 mm in diameter. In side branches <2.5 mm, the stent should be avoided if possible. Of course there are occasional exceptions, and we have at times performed double stenting with a 2.25-mm stent, particularly when the side branch is long with a somewhat large territory of distribution. Compared with bare-metal stenting, we are more liberal in the use of a stent in small branch when we are implanting a drug-eluting stent which may guarantee minimal late loss. In some cases, stenting of the side branch may be required if, during the dilatation, the side branch occludes, dissects, or has an impaired flow.

WHEN TO PERFORM ATHERECTOMY

When dealing with drug-eluting stents, many people may consider this question almost inappropriate because we should expect optimal outcome just with stent implantation. Unfortunately, this is not always the end result, and in about 20% of the cases we see some recurrence at the ostium of the side branch. It is important to mention that many of these recurrences are clinically silent and are not associated with any demonstrable ischemia. For all these reasons, it becomes difficult sometimes to suggest a more complex associated procedure such as directional atherectomy.

At the present time, we have no specific suggestions regarding when to use atherectomy with either of the two devices available (Atherocath, Guidant, or Silverhawk, Foxhollow), in the context of drug-eluting stent implantation. Most of the time, the decision is made by the operator on the basis of technical suitability, large plaque burden, or personal preference. We doubt whether the literature will give us any new important information to answer this question.

TECHNIQUES FOR STENTING BIFURCATIONAL LESIONS

A classification of bifurcational lesions has been recently proposed by Safian[1] (Figure 1), which is a minor change from a prior scheme proposed by Lefevre.[2] The following are some different techniques of stent implantation in bifurcations that were actually performed in our laboratory.[3–10]

The standard approach: stenting the main branch and dilating the side branch through the struts

The easiest way to stent a bifurcation is to stent the main branch covering the ostium of the side branch. However, several precautions should be considered. Side branches, which are not significantly compromised (angiographic diameter stenosis ≤50%) might not need to be dilated. When there is a lumen compromise (>50%) of a small side branch (<2.0 mm) with reasonable thrombolysis in myocardial infarction (TIMI) flow and no signs of ischemia, the operator should resist the temptation to do anything other than to call the case finished. It is known that an excellent long-term patency rate is present when a side branch is even modestly patent at the end of the stenting procedure on the major branch.[11,12]

When necessary, the struts of most stents are easily crossed with a wire. The bifurcation is frequently approached with advancement of two wires (one in the main branch and the other in the side branch). The stent is advanced in the main

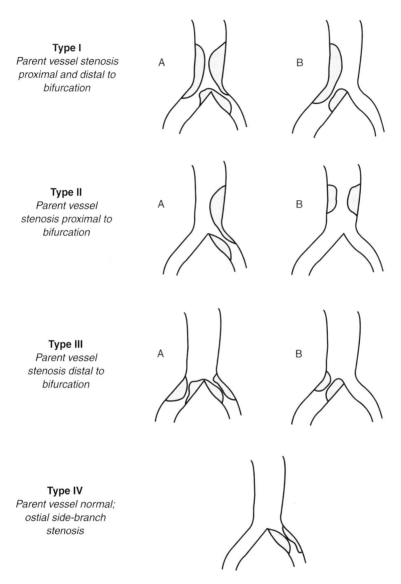

Type I
Parent vessel stenosis proximal and distal to bifurcation

Type II
Parent vessel stenosis proximal to bifurcation

Type III
Parent vessel stenosis distal to bifurcation

Type IV
Parent vessel normal; ostial side-branch stenosis

Figure 1   Schematic presentation of bifurcation types. A: side branch involved; B: side branch normal

branch and implanted, trapping the side-branch wire underneath the struts. It is important to inflate the stent at low pressure in order to facilitate removal of the wire below the stent struts. The wire in the side branch is useful for directing the second wire, which is now advanced through the stent struts into the side branch. We frequently use the wire that is in the main vessel for advancement into the side branch. Following successful advancement of this wire into the side branch, the wire trapped below the stent struts is now removed and advanced in the main branch. If all the above maneuvers are difficult, a new wire needs to be used to access the side branch. The new wire should be shaped to an angle of approximately 90°, and after the tip is engaged within the struts at the origin of the side branch, a slight backward movement with careful steering allows crossing into the side branch. In case of no success, reshaping of the tip with a wider, >90° curve, should be attempted. Hydrophilic-coated wires (Pilot 50 or 150, Guidant) might find less friction in crossing the struts, or an intermediate type of stiffer wire may facilitate engagement into the ostium of side branch, but there will be an increased risk of dissecting the side branch. In the case of no success, a 1.5-mm or 2.0-mm fixed-wire balloon (Ace or Pivot, Boston Scientific) or a double-lumen open-ended catheter (Multifunctional Probing Catheter, Boston Scientific) can be advanced close to the origin of the side branch to increase the support of the wire crossing the struts. The fact that the probing catheter is advanced over the wire coaxial to the stent deployed in the main branch will also prevent the second wire from engaging below the struts of the main-branch stent.

After wire crossing, a balloon needs to be advanced into the side branch. This can be very easy, but sometimes the use of new, unexpanded, low-diameter and low-profile balloons is necessary. Generally, the balloon should not be advanced completely into the side branch for inflation because this increases the risk of balloon entrapment. The inflation pressure should also be kept well under the rated burst pressure because balloon rupture within a stent strut can also cause balloon entrapment.

An alternative to crossing the stent strut can be a balloon with a fixed wire. The fixed wire serves as a transition between wire and balloon with a low profile that preserves optimal pushability, and allows for comfortable strut crossing. Furthermore, this method is quick, only one device needs to be inserted, and the low-profile device accommodates a normal balloon found in 6-Fr guide-catheters. Finally, kissing balloon inflations in both the stented main branch and in the side branch should liberally be performed because stent deformation following side-branch dilatation might have occurred.

The modified T-stent technique

This technique can be best employed when the side branch originates with an angle of 90° (or close to 90°)[4,7] (Figure 2). If the operator accepts some overlap between the stents, the modified T-technique can be used in almost any bifurcation for which two stents need to be implanted. Both branches are wired and alternatively dilated. A first stent is advanced into the side branch but not expanded, and a second stent is advanced into the main branch, extending distally and proximally to the ostium of the side branch. Then, the first stent is carefully retracted to protrude slightly from the ostium of the side branch into the main branch. The amount of protrusion into the main branch depends on the angle between main and side branch. For side branches

Step 1: Wire and dilate both branches

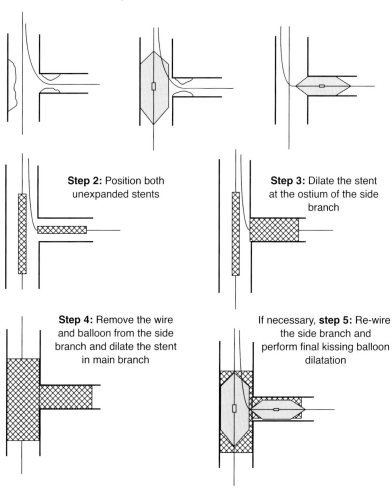

Step 2: Position both unexpanded stents

Step 3: Dilate the stent at the ostium of the side branch

Step 4: Remove the wire and balloon from the side branch and dilate the stent in main branch

If necessary, **step 5:** Re-wire the side branch and perform final kissing balloon dilatation

Figure 2 The modified T-stenting technique

with an angle of origin from the main branch that is close to 90°, the protrusion needs to be minimal. For side branches with a smaller angle (V-origin), it is necessary to have more protrusion into the main branch in order to completely cover the carina. When the side-branch stent is appropriately positioned, the balloon is inflated and the stent is deployed. We found that the side-branch stent is in a proper position when its proximal balloon marker lies in the same line as the two balloon markers of the stent present in the main branch.

Following deployment of the side-branch stent, the balloon is removed, and a test injection is made to ensure that there is no distal dissection. This is the time to treat any residual distal dissection. In case this unlikely event occurs, the operator may need to advance an additional short stent into the side branch before removing the wire. Following documentation of a good flow and angiographic result in the side branch, the wire is removed. Then the stent in the main branch is expanded and the side branch is rewired. This maneuver can be tedious at times, and different technical tricks may be necessary (Intermediate wire, or Pivot balloon, Boston Scientific). Following side-branch rewiring, the side-branch stent is re-dilated at its proximal part with a balloon sized to the side-branch diameter. In case of difficulties, the first dilatation may require a 1.5-mm balloon. Final kissing balloon inflation is performed at a medium pressure (8 atm) with two balloons sized to the diameter of the distal end of the stent in each branch.

This technique is reasonably safe because both stents are positioned before inflation, thereby abolishing the difficulties of crossing a second stent (T-technique). The major disadvantages of this technique are: recrossing into the side branch may be complex; and when the origin of the side branch is close to a V, more stent struts protruding into the main branch will need to be crushed against one side of the main branch.

Some operators use a variation of this technique to stent ostial side-branch lesions. In this situation, instead of placing a stent in the main branch, a simple balloon catheter is positioned in the main branch to better locate the exact position of the ostium of the side branch and to perform low-pressure inflation in the main branch if needed.

When the T-technique is used with drug-eluting stents, there is almost always the risk of leaving the ostium of the side branch not fully covered by stent struts and without any drug delivered at the ostium.

Basically, the modified T-stenting technique is the preamble to the crush technique. The way in which we discussed the modified T-stenting technique for bifurcations, with an acute angle suggesting some protrusion of the side-branch stent in the main branch, is basically the crush technique.

'Crush' stenting technique

The use of drug-eluting stents significantly reduced the incidence of angiographic restenosis in the Bifurcations Study (An Evaluation of the Sirolimus-coated Bx Velocity Stent in the Treatment of Patients with True Bifurcation Lesions), but also revealed the prevailing occurrence of restenosis at the ostium of the side branch.[13] Incomplete coverage of the ostium of the side branch was the most probable cause of restenosis. To overcome that problem, we designed a new technique for stenting bifurcational lesions: modified T-stenting with 'crush'.[14]

The crush technique is presented in Figure 3. Both branches are wired and alternatively dilated. A first stent is advanced into the side branch but not expanded, and a second stent is advanced into the main branch to fully cover the bifurcation. The side-branch stent is retracted into the main branch for 2–3 mm. The proximal

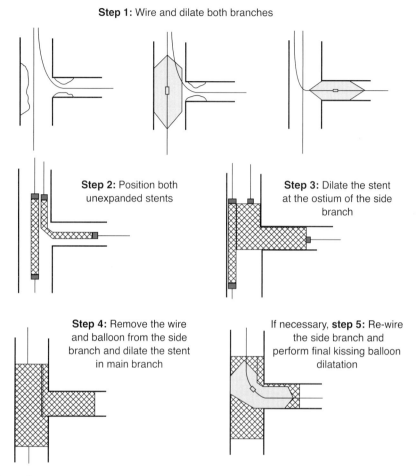

Step 1: Wire and dilate both branches

Step 2: Position both unexpanded stents

Step 3: Dilate the stent at the ostium of the side branch

Step 4: Remove the wire and balloon from the side branch and dilate the stent in main branch

If necessary, **step 5:** Re-wire the side branch and perform final kissing balloon dilatation

Figure 3   The crush stenting technique

marker of the side-branch stent must be situated in the main branch at a distance of few millimeters proximally to the carina of the bifurcation. The stent in the side branch will protrude in the main branch in a similar fashion to the procedure employed by the operator when performing the culottes technique,[6] except that the protrusion should be kept minimal to the amount necessary to fully cover the ostium of the side branch. In this way, the ostium of the side branch is ensured to be circumferentially covered with stent struts. It is important to position the stent in the main branch so that it will cover the entire lesion in this branch. It is also important to ensure that the main-branch stent is in the appropriate position, because following expansion of the stent in the side branch, it may be difficult to move and reposition the stent in the main branch in any direction.

When the side-branch stent is appropriately positioned, the balloon is inflated and the stent is deployed. After stent implantation, the proximal part of this stent will clearly protrude in the main vessel. The delivery balloon is removed from the side branch and a contrast injection is performed to ensure that no distal dissection is present and no additional stents are needed in the side branch. It is possible at this time to advance another stent in the side branch in case it is needed. The wire is then removed from the side branch. Then, the stent in the main branch is expanded. During balloon inflation and stent implantation in the main branch, the protruding struts of the stent implanted in the side branch are crushed against the wall of the main vessel. In this way, there are no floating struts; instead there are three layers of struts in the proximal part of the bifurcation and near the ostium of the side branch. In our initial experience, we evaluated the result in multiple projections, and the procedure was considered complete if angiographically acceptable. Currently, we always recross towards the side branch and perform first high-pressure balloon inflation towards the side branch and finally a kissing balloon inflation. Another recent technical refinement has been the frequent usage of a short (6-mm-long) cutting balloon to prepare the ostium of the side branch before stent delivery. If necessary, following kissing inflation, an additional stent can also be advanced in the side branch to treat an overlooked distal dissection.

Variations of the crush technique

Provisional crush (reverse crush) (side-branch stent crushed by a balloon)   The main purpose of performing the reverse crush is to allow an opportunity for provisional side-branch stenting. The reverse crush can be performed utilizing a 6-Fr guiding catheter. The technique is described as follows.

Step one: a stent is deployed in the main branch, and balloon dilatation with kissing inflation towards the side branch is performed. It is assumed that the result at the ostium or at the proximal segment of the side branch will be such that the operator will decide to deploy a stent at this site.

Step two: a second stent is advanced into the side branch and left in position without being deployed.

Step three: a balloon sized according to the diameter of the main branch is advanced in the main branch and positioned at the level of the bifurcation, paying attention to stay inside the stent previously deployed in the main branch.

Step four: the stent in the side branch is retracted about 2 3 mm into the main branch and deployed, the deploying balloon is removed, and an angiogram is obtained to verify no distal dissection or distal stent is needed. If such is the case, the wire from the side branch is removed, and the balloon in the main branch is inflated at high pressure (≥ 12 atm).

The others steps are similar to those described for the crush technique and involve recrossing into the side branch to perform side-branch dilatation and final kissing.

Inverted crush (side-branch stent crushes the main-branch stent)

The key element of this technique is to crush the main-branch stent with the side-branch stent rather than the other way around. This approach should be considered when the two branches are of similar size and when the angle of origin of the side branch from the main branch is unfavorable for recrossing. There are various reasons for performing this technique: the step which involves recrossing the stents following deployment of both stents is easier owing to the fact that recrossing goes in the direction of the main branch which is usually less angulated; and if the main branch has diffuse disease proximally and distally to the bifurcation, two stents can treat both the bifurcations and the proximal and distal disease. (This goal is accomplished by extending the use of the long stent: the one of the side branch is two thirds of its length in the main branch, and the one in the main branch is two thirds of its length distal to the bifurcations.)

The main limitation of this technique is due to the fact that the stent in the diagonal branch will be used to stent a significant segment of the main branch. This is not a problem if the size of the main branch is ≤ 3 mm. An 8-Fr guiding catheter is needed to perform the inverted crush technique. The technique is described as follows.

Step one: step one is the same as with the standard crush technique.

Step two: a stent is advanced in the main branch distally to the bifurcation. A second stent is advanced in the side branch as much as needed to cover the diseased segment in the side branch and as much as needed to cover the diseased segment in the main branch. (The stent length is chosen according to the total length of the diseased segment proximal to the bifurcation in the main branch and distal to the bifurcation in the side branch.) The main-branch stent (the one which completely lies in the main branch and which is more distally located) is pulled back a few millimeters proximally to the bifurcation. The length of this stent is chosen according to the length of the diseased segment distally to the bifurcation. We always try to minimize the amount of overlap or crush to what is needed to ensure proper coverage of the ostium.

Step three: the stent which fully lies in the main branch (the most distal one) is deployed. The balloon is removed and angiography is performed to verify the result. The wire is then pulled back and the other stent is deployed, usually at ≥ 12 atm.

Step four: the balloon which deployed the stent in the side branch is pulled back slightly proximally to the bifurcation, and the wire (which has been left in the balloon) is advanced through the stent's struts into the distal segment of the main vessel. This maneuver is usually easier because the angle is more favorable, and this is one important reason for performing this technique. Following wiring of the distal main branch, the balloon on this wire is removed (we will not try to use this balloon to recross into the distal segment). A wire is then advanced into the proximal stent and towards the side branch. It is important to pay attention not to go underneath the stent struts, particularly because the proximal stent may be under-dilated. This maneuver is usually not complex owing to the fact that the stent goes into that direction.

Step five: a balloon sized according to the distal segment of the main branch is advanced over the bifurcation into the distal stent, and a balloon sized according to the proximal segment is used to fully dilate the proximal segment of the stent.

Step six: a final kissing (main branch towards side branch and main branch distal and proximal to the bifurcation) is performed again at 8 atm, or lower if there is a gross mismatching between the proximal (to the bifurcation) main-branch segment and the side branch. In the case of gross mismatching and of concerns of overdilatation of the side branch, the final kissing will need to be performed with a smaller balloon (the balloon will always protrude in the side branch). This is the reason why we prefer not to use this technique when there is a large difference in diameter between the main branch and the side branch.

The inverted crush has been introduced recently, and we are now evaluating whether any additional advantage in terms of restenosis is gained when utilizing this technique.

Step crushing (side-branch stent crushed by the main-branch stent)   The main reason for implementing this technique is to perform the standard crush technique utilizing a 6-Fr guiding catheter. Operators who perform the radial approach may be particularly interested in this technique. The final result is basically similar to the one obtained with the standard crush technique, the only difference being that each stent is advanced and deployed separately in order to use a 6-Fr guide. As mentioned earlier, the need for a 6-Fr guide is the only reason for utilizing this technique. The technique is described as follows.

Step one: step one is the same as with the standard crush technique.

Step two: a stent is advanced in the side branch protruding into the main branch a few millimeters. A balloon (Maverick, Boston Scientific) is advanced in the main branch over the bifurcation.

Step three: the stent in the side branch is deployed, the balloon removed, an angio is performed, and if the result is adequate the wire is also removed. The main branch balloon is then inflated (to crush the protruding side branch stent) and removed.

Step four: a stent is advanced in the main branch and deployed (usually at ≥ 12 atm).

The next steps are similar to the crush technique and involve recrossing into the side branch, side-branch stent dilatation, and final kissing balloon dilatation.

The T-stenting technique

This technique is performed by placing the first stent in the main branch and then by wiring the side branch (Figure 4).[7–9] Following side-branch access through the deployed stent, the struts of the main-branch stent are dilated towards the side branch, and then a second stent is advanced into the side branch. Again, as in the modified T-technique, the operator will decide how much the stent in the side branch will protrude into the main branch. Following dilatation of the side-branch stent, inflation is performed in the main branch and then a final kissing inflation.

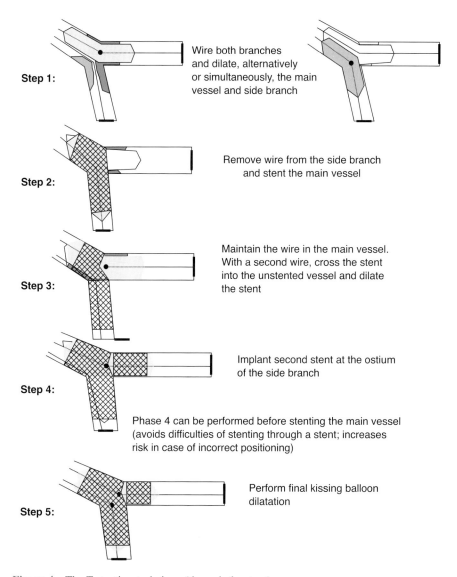

Step 1: Wire both branches and dilate, alternatively or simultaneously, the main vessel and side branch

Step 2: Remove wire from the side branch and stent the main vessel

Step 3: Maintain the wire in the main vessel. With a second wire, cross the stent into the unstented vessel and dilate the stent

Step 4: Implant second stent at the ostium of the side branch

Phase 4 can be performed before stenting the main vessel (avoids difficulties of stenting through a stent; increases risk in case of incorrect positioning)

Step 5: Perform final kissing balloon dilatation

Figure 4 The T-stenting technique (through the stent)

The V-stenting technique

This is a 'kissing stents' technique suitable for bifurcations of two large side branches with a large diameter of the vessel proximal to the bifurcation. As the name implies, this technique is best suited for branches which originate with a narrow angle ($<70°$, Figure 5).

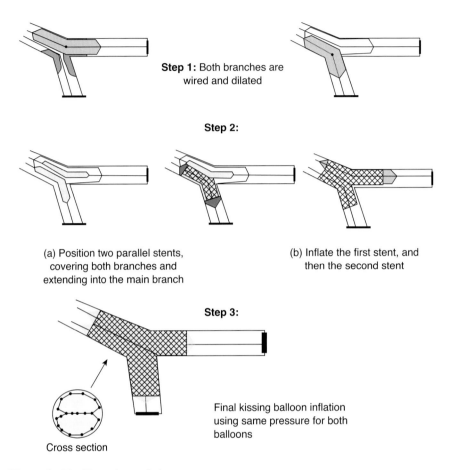

Step 1: Both branches are wired and dilated

Step 2:

(a) Position two parallel stents, covering both branches and extending into the main branch

(b) Inflate the first stent, and then the second stent

Step 3:

Final kissing balloon inflation using same pressure for both balloons

Cross section

Figure 5   The V-stenting technique

Both branches are wired and alternatively predilated. Subsequently, the two unexpanded stents are positioned close to the ostium of the branches with a slight abutment into the main vessel. It is better to expand the two stents alternatively, in order to avoid dislodgment of one balloon during simultaneous inflations. High-pressure inflation with short balloons might be performed alternatively, but the final inflation should be a simultaneous ('kissing'), using the same pressure and balloons sized according to the diameter of the two branches.

Using this technique, a metallic neo-carina is created within the vessel proximal to the bifurcation. Theoretical concerns of an increased risk of thrombosis owing to the neo-carina have not been confirmed in our experience. This technique is simple and safe because access to both branches is always maintained. The lesion coverage is also complete. However, when compared with the 'culottes' technique, the V-technique has more limited applications and is suited only for very large branches with a narrow angle of origin. Quick performance, easy execution, and safety are the major advantages of the V-technique. Dr S. Sharma from Mount Sinai Hospital in New York is popularizing the V-technique with the Cypher stent to be employed in most of the bifurcations. The follow-up results are eagerly awaited in order to evaluate the possible come back of this approach.

The 'culottes' stenting technique

This 'culottes' stent technique was first described by Chevalier *et al.*[6] and is, in our view, the most elegant method for stenting both branches of a bifurcation. The technique is described in Figure 6. The culottes technique should only be utilized with stents that do not have a closed-cell design (Taxus, Boston Scientific) or stents with cells that can be opened to a diameter large enough to fully appose the open cell to the wall of the main branch and give an appropriate access to the main and side branch (Cypher, Cordis) when the branch is ≤3 mm. Both branches are wired and pre-dilated alternatively; subsequently, the wire is removed from the straighter branch and the more angulated branch is stented. Obviously, if an important dissection or occlusion occurs in one branch, this branch should be stented first because wire removal might be risky. Following this step, the wire is removed from the stented branch and used to rewire the branch not yet stented. This step is performed by advancing the wire through the struts of the stent already deployed. The stent struts should now be dilated toward the un-stented branch. In case the balloon does not cross, a small-diameter (1.5 mm) low-profile balloon can be used. Then, a second stent is advanced and expanded into the un-stented branch maintaining the proximal part of the stent within the previous deployed stent. Finally, the first stented branch is re-wired and final kissing balloon inflation is performed.

With this technique, the vessel proximal to the bifurcation is partially covered by two overlapping stents, and each branch is covered by a single stent. This technique can also be used when the initial plan was to stent only one vessel and the result on the second branch deteriorated to a level that suggested the stenting of this branch too. A possible problem associated with the performance of the culottes technique is that, at the time of deployment of the stent in the most angulated branch (usually the side branch), the operator needs to remove the wire from the main branch, and then he needs to recross again through the stent's struts towards the main branch. Finally, he needs to recross again towards the side branch, this time through a double layer of struts.

We used this technique several times with the Taxus stent, and hitherto we have not encountered any problems related to double dosage of the drug at the site of overlap.

The Y-stenting technique

This technique implies the use of multiple stents and was probably the first technique ever used for true bifurcation stenting.[15,16] The technique can be summarized

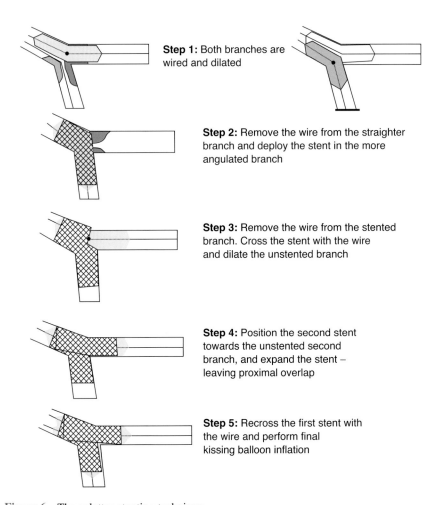

Step 1: Both branches are wired and dilated

Step 2: Remove the wire from the straighter branch and deploy the stent in the more angulated branch

Step 3: Remove the wire from the stented branch. Cross the stent with the wire and dilate the unstented branch

Step 4: Position the second stent towards the unstented second branch, and expand the stent – leaving proximal overlap

Step 5: Recross the first stent with the wire and perform final kissing balloon inflation

Figure 6   The culottes stenting technique

in three steps (Figure 7): both branches are wired and predilated, a stent is deployed and expanded at the ostium of each branch with kissing dilatations (separate inflations), and a proximal stent is crimped on two balloons leaving the distal part of the balloons uncovered from the stent. The stent is then advanced on the two wires, until the distal part of both balloons enters the ostia of the vessel with the previously deployed stents. This proximal stent is deployed, inflating both balloons as close as possible to the carina. Finally, kissing balloon inflation within the three stents is performed.

The advantage of this technique is that wire access to both branches is always maintained. The lesion coverage, however, may not be perfect. This is a relatively

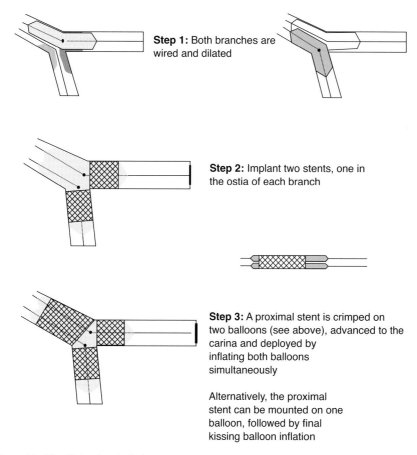

Step 1: Both branches are wired and dilated

Step 2: Implant two stents, one in the ostia of each branch

Step 3: A proximal stent is crimped on two balloons (see above), advanced to the carina and deployed by inflating both balloons simultaneously

Alternatively, the proximal stent can be mounted on one balloon, followed by final kissing balloon inflation

Figure 7 The Y-stenting technique

complex technique which requires three stents and very careful wire handling to prevent wire crossing. An alternative and more contemporary approach which does not require manual crimping of a stent on two balloons, is to deploy the proximal stent on a single balloon after removal of the wire from one branch. This branch is then re-wired and final kissing balloon inflations are performed.

'Skirt' technique

A more recent technique for dealing with a bifurcational lesion without stenting the side branch, but maintaining the largest possible patency of the proximal part of the bifurcation ('inflow'), can be applied when the disease involves only the proximal portion of the bifurcation (Figure 8). Both branches are predilated using the

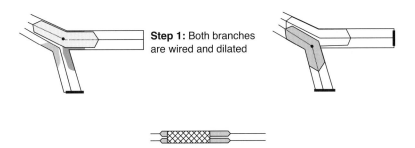

Step 1: Both branches are wired and dilated

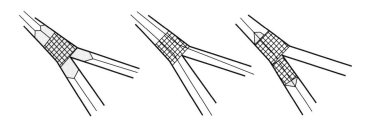

Step 2: A stent is crimped on two balloons, leaving the distal portions of the balloons uncovered ('stent sandwich')

Step 3: Advance the balloons on both wires until the stent hits the carina and deploy the stent by inflating both balloons

If necessary, a distal stent can be implanted in the main branch, slightly overlapping the proximal stent

Figure 8   Creating a proximal funnel technique (the skirt technique)

double-wire technique. A stent is crimped on two balloons of appropriate diameter according to the size of the two branches. The stent (about half the length of the balloons) 'sandwiches' both balloons, leaving their distal portions uncovered. The two balloons are advanced on the two wires until the stent hits the carina and the stent is deployed. The distal part of the stent will open towards both branches, creating a funnel just proximal to the bifurcation. A distal stent in any of the two branches could be subsequently implanted if necessary.

This technique is relatively easy to perform and does not commit to side-branch stenting. The presence of disease just proximal to small side branches (≤ 3.0 mm) is the main consideration in using this approach. Similar to the Y-technique, this approach needs manual crimping of the stent on two balloons, and today it is of only historical value.

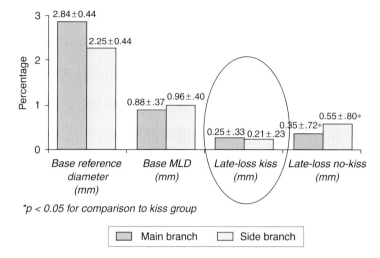

Figure 9 Six-month quantitative coronary angiography results of patients treated with the crush technique

Stent distortion during side-branch dilatation

A study of side-branch dilatation in animal coronaries[17] showed the presence of an important distortion of the Palmaz-Schatz stent when a balloon is dilated through a strut and a lesser distortion when dilated at the articulation site. Ormiston *et al.*[18] simulated a dilatation of a side branch at an angle of 45° in a Plexiglas model. They evaluated the diameter of the created side lumen and the distortion of the stent in the main vessel distal to the inflated side branch in terms of distal diameter stenosis. The occurrence of a distal distortion following dilatation into the side branch underlines the importance of performing a kissing inflation of the bifurcation.

Importance of final kissing when two stents are used

Our experience of bifurcational stenting utilizing two stents has taught us how important it is to perform two steps: high-pressure inflation in the side branch following wire recrossing and final kissing inflation, usually at 8 atm.

The restenosis rate at the ostium of the side branch decreased from 25% when two drug-eluting stents are implanted without final kissing to less than 10% when final kissing is used. Preliminary results of our experience with the crush technique, performed with the Cypher stent and confronting the procedures performed without final kissing to the ones with final kissing, are presented in Figures 9 and 10, and Table 2.

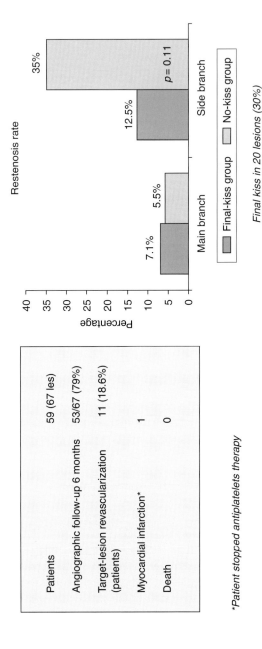

*Patient stopped antiplatelets therapy

Figure 10   Six-month clinical outcome of patients treated with the crush technique

Table 2   Immediate outcome of patients treated with the crush technique

Patients	59
Bifurcational lesion*	67
True bifurcational	47 (71%)
Final kissing	20 (30%)
Q-MI	4 (6.7%)
Death	0

*Left main lesions were excluded

CONCLUSIONS

The most important issue when performing bifurcational stenting is to decide whether two stents or one stent should be used. When possible, the operator should propose a strategy of stent implantation only in the main branch.

Bifurcational stenting demands an appropriate balance between procedural risk and long-term results in achieving an optimal outcome. Coronary stenting has the potential to achieve superb immediate results, which all too frequently are not maintained at the follow-up. The operator should always keep this paradox in mind.

The availability of drug-eluting stents have made a significant improvement in the long-term results of bifurcational stenting.[13] We can say that restenosis at the main branch has been almost eliminated, and restenosis at the side branch has been reduced by 50%.

It may be possible that use of some new techniques for better covering the ostium of the side branch, particularly following appropriate side-branch pre-dilatations may further reduce the recurrence at this site.

REFERENCES

1. Safian RD. Bifurcation Lesions. Royal Oak: Physicians' Press; 2001
2. Lefevre T, Louvard Y, Morice MC, et al. Stenting of bifurcation lesions: classification, treatments, and results. Catheter Cardiovasc Interv 2000; 49: 274–83
3. Colombo A, Gaglione A, Nakamura S, Finci L. 'Kissing' stents for bifurcational coronary lesion. Cathet Cardiovasc Diagn 1993; 30: 327–30
4. Nakamura S, Hall P, Maiello L, Colombo A. Techniques for Palmaz-Schatz stent deployment in lesions with a large side branch. Cathet Cardiovasc Diagn 1995; 34: 353–61
5. Kobayashi Y, Colombo A, Akiyama T, et al. Modified 'T' stenting: a technique for kissing stents in bifurcational coronary lesion. Cathet Cardiovasc Diagn 1998; 43: 323–6
6. Chevalier B, Glatt B, Royer T, Guyon P. Placement of coronary stents in bifurcation lesions by the 'culotte' technique. Am J Cardiol 1998; 82: 943–9
7. Carrie D, Karouny E, Chouairi S, Puel J. 'T'-shaped stent placement: a technique for the treatment of dissected bifurcation lesions. Cathet Cardiovasc Diagn 1996; 37: 311–3

8. Anzuini A, Briguori C, Rosanio S, et al. Immediate and long-term clinical and angiographic results from Wiktor stent treatment for true bifurcation narrowings. Am J Cardiol 2001; 88: 1246–50

9. Sheiban I, Albiero R, Marsico F, et al. Immediate and long-term results of 'T' stenting for bifurcation coronary lesions. Am J Cardiol 2000; 85: 1141–4, A9

10. Di Mario C, Airoldi F, Reimers B, et al. Bifurcational stenting. Semin Interv Cardiol 1998; 3: 65–76

11. Fischman DL, Savage MP, Leon MB, et al. Fate of lesion-related side branches after coronary artery stenting. J Am Coll Cardiol 1993; 22: 1641–6

12. Pan M, Medina A, Suarez de Lezo J, et al. Follow-up patency of side branches covered by intracoronary Palmaz-Schatz stent. Am Heart J 1995; 129: 436–40

13. Colombo A, Moses JW, Morice MC, et al. Randomized study to evaluate sirolimus-eluting stents implanted at coronary bifurcation lesions. Circulation 2004; 109: 1244–9

14. Colombo A, Stankovic G, Orlic D, et al. Modified T-stenting technique with crushing for bifurcation lesions: Immediate results and 30-day outcome. Catheter Cardiovasc Interv 2003; 60: 145–51

15. Fort S, Lazzam C, Schwartz L. Coronary 'Y' stenting: a technique for angioplasty of bifurcation stenoses. Can J Cardiol 1996; 12: 678–82

16. Baim DS. Is birfucation stenting the answer? Cathet Cardiovasc Diagn 1996; 37: 314–6

17. Pomerantz RM, Ling FS. Distortion of Palmaz-Schatz stent geometry following side-branch balloon dilation through the stent in a rabbit model. Cathet Cardiovasc Diagn 1997; 40: 422–6

18. Ormiston JA, Webster MW, Ruygrok PN, et al. Stent deformation following simulated side-branch dilatation: a comparison of five stent designs. Catheter Cardiovasc Interv 1999; 47: 258–64

Lessons from the literature

Goran Stankovic MD

INTRODUCTION

Coronary bifurcations are at high risk for the development of atherosclerotic plaque due to turbulent flow and low shear stress.[1–4] Since the introduction of percutaneous coronary revascularization, lesions situated at bifurcations have become one of the most intriguing and challenging subsets and, in experienced centers, account for 12–18% of coronary angioplasty procedures.[5–9] Historical data suggest that treatment of bifurcational lesions is associated with decreased success and increased complication rates compared with non-bifurcational lesions.[10] The most common problems that we face in bifurcation treatment are: side-branch (SB) access; SB compromise (deterioration or SB occlusion – 'snow-plough' effect); incomplete coverage of the SB ostium with the stent; stent distortion; and high rates of restenosis (slide 2).[8,9]

Angulation and morphology

Bifurcational lesions are classified according to the angulation of the bifurcation and plaque burden (slide 3).[8,9] These determine ease of access to side branch, plaque shift and hence preferred treatment strategies.

On the basis of angulation, lesions are classified as Y-shaped (side-branch and main-branch angulation < 70°) or T-shaped (side-branch and main-branch angulation > 70°). In Y-shaped lesions, access to the side branch is easy, but there is significant plaque shift during PCI. The converse holds true for T-shaped lesions.

Location of the plaque burden is also crucial, and four types of lesions have been described: *Type I lesion* ('true bifurcation') – disease involves the main branch both proximal and distal to the side branch, as well as the ostium of the side branch. *Type II lesion* – disease involves the main branch at the bifurcation site, but not the ostium of the side branch. *Type III lesion* – disease involves primarily the main branch immediately proximal to the origin of an unobstructed side branch. *Type IV lesion* – disease is located at the ostium of each branch with sparing of the proximal section of the bifurcation, with two subtypes: *Type IVa,* where there is only a main-branch ostial lesion distal to the bifurcation and *Type IVb,* where the lesion involves only the ostium of the side branch. For all the 'pseudobifurcational' lesions (types II-IV), treating the proximal lesion often results in plaque shift into the side branch, converting the original lesion into a bifurcational lesion.

A difficult challenge

Treatment of bifurcational lesions with balloon angioplasty has been a difficult challenge and was associated with a low procedural success and high complication and restenosis rates despite refinement of the technique using kissing balloon inflation (slide 4).[1,11–15] Ineffective lumen expansion in both the main vessel and the side branch due to plaque shift and lesion recoil can frequently be observed.[11,16–20] Treatment of bifurcations with directional atherectomy has been shown to improve the procedural outcome, but the incidence of restenosis has remained high.[21–24] Despite an intuitive perception that atherectomy may eliminate or lessen plaque shift in bifurcational lesions, there are no reports documenting this advantage.

Coronary stents reduce lesion recoil by achieving effective lumen scaffolding (slide 5).[25,26] However, coronary stents may also compromise side branches,[17,27–30] thereby increasing the incidence of procedural complications in cases of bifurcational stenting.

Several techniques have been proposed for stenting bifurcational lesions.[31–41]

Louvard *et al.* recently summarized all stenting techniques (slide 6) as:

- *Type A treatment* – placement of a stent at the side-branch ostium followed by placement of another stent in the main branch covering the ostium of the side branch
- *Type B treatment* – stenting of the main branch followed by stenting of the side branch at the ostium level through the struts of the main-branch stent
- *Type C treatment* – this technique is known as the 'culottes' or 'trousers' technique or, in some instances, as the Y-technique. It consists of implanting a first stent from the proximal to the distal segment of the main branch, jailing the side-branch ostium. A second stent is then placed from the proximal main branch towards the side branch while jailing the ostium of the distal main branch. This results in a double layer of stents in the proximal part of the main branch
- *Type D treatment* – this strategy consists of placing two stents at the level of the ostia, followed by implantation of another stent in the proximal segment if necessary. This technique is also known as the Y-implantation technique

The impact of introduction of new interventional techniques such as atherectomy or early-generation coronary stents on procedural and the 1-year clinical outcome of patients with bifurcational lesions were assessed in a large registry (NHLBI dynamic registry) (slide 7).[10] The authors concluded that despite the widespread use of newer percutaneous devices, the treatment of bifurcational lesions remains difficult and is associated with decreased success and increased complication rates compared with nonbifurcational lesions. Patients with bifurcational lesions had lower angiographic success, a higher rate of SB occlusion, and a higher rate of in-hospital and 1-year major adverse cardiac events (MACE).

Slide 8 addresses the learning curve for bifurcational stenting. The strategy of systematic coronary stenting in bifurcational lesions involving a side branch ≥ 2.2 mm in diameter was prospectively evaluated in a single-center observational study during a 35-month inclusion period.[6] Analysis of the 7-month outcome according to two study periods (period I, 1 January 1996 to 31 August 1997, 182 patients; period II, 1 September 1997 to 30 June 1998, 127 patients) showed that the target-vessel revascularization (TVR) rate decreased from 20.6 to 13.8% ($p = 0.04$) and the MACE rate from 29.2 to 17.1% ($p < 0.01$) in period I and II, respectively. This was associated, by univariate analysis, with an increasing use of tubular stents deployed in the main branch (94.2 vs. 59.1%, $p < 0.001$) and kissing balloon inflation after coronary stenting (75.4 vs. 18.1%, $p < 0.001$). The authors concluded that in-hospital and follow-up results are influenced not only by the learning curve but also by the use of tubular stents in the main branch and final kissing balloon inflation.

Slide 9 deals with an important issue with bifurcational lesions: two stents versus one stent. There are no large prospective randomized trials addressing long-term clinical outcome with the use of stent versus balloon dilatation or surgery and of different stenting techniques in patients requiring PCI for bifurcational lesions. The majority of the information is based on reports from a number of registries and retrospective data.

Several authors have evaluated two different techniques of stent placement in bifurcational lesions, stenting both branches versus stenting main branch only with SB angioplasty. Although the results are variable, most reports demonstrate no added advantage in stenting both the parent vessel as well as the side branch. Yamashita *et al.* reported that between March 1993 and April 1999, a total of 92 patients with bifurcational lesions were treated with two strategies: stenting both vessels (group B, $n = 53$) or stenting the parent vessel and performing balloon angioplasty of the side branch (group P, $n = 39$).[42] Stent placement on both branches resulted in a lower residual stenosis in the side branch, and acute procedural success was similar in the two groups (group B: 87% vs. Group P: 92%). In-hospital MACE occurred only in group B (13% vs. 0%, $p < 0.05$). At the 6-month follow-up, the angiographic restenosis rate (group B: 62% vs. Group P: 48%) and the target-lesion revascularization rate (38% vs. 36%, respectively) were similar in the two groups. There was no difference in the incidence of 6-month total MACE (51% vs. 38%). The authors concluded that for the treatment of true bifurcational lesions, a complex strategy of stenting both vessels provided no advantage in terms of procedural success and late outcome compared with a simpler strategy of stenting only the parent vessel.

A similar design study was published by Al Suwaidi *et al.* (slide 10)[43] Between October 1993 and November 1998, 131 patients with bifurcational lesions treated with stents were divided into two groups; Group (Gp) 1 included 77 patients treated with a stent in one branch and percutaneous transluminal coronary angioplasty (PTCA) (with or without atherectomy) in the side branch, and Gp 2 included

54 patients who underwent stent deployment in both branches. The Gp 2 patients were subsequently divided into two subgroups depending on the technique of stent deployment. Gp 2a included 19 patients who underwent Y-stenting, and Gp 2b included 33 patients who underwent T-stenting. Procedural success rates were comparable in both groups (89.5–97.4%). After 1-year follow-up, no significant differences were seen in the frequency of MACE (death, MI, or repeat revascularization) between Gp 1 and Gp 2. Adverse cardiac events were higher with Y-stenting compared with T-stenting (86.3% vs. 30.4%, $p=0.004$). The author concluded that stenting of both branches offers no advantage over stenting one branch and performing balloon angioplasty of the other branch.

The value of provisional versus systematic stenting of both branches in patients with true bifurcational lesions was addressed by Dr Lefevre at the 2002 ESC meeting. (slide 11)[44] Among 936 bifurcational lesions consecutively included, 474 (51%) were type 1. Systematic T-stenting, stenting the side branch first (Type A treatment) was used in 19% of cases. Stenting of the main branch with provisional T-stenting of the side branch (Type B) was used in 74% of cases, 'culottes' stenting (type C) in 3% of cases and others in 4%. The authors concluded that provisional T-stenting of the side branch is the least time-consuming strategy associated with a lower rate of 7-month MACE (17% vs. 29%) and TVR (13% vs. 23%) compared with other strategies.

At the same meeting, Dr Lefevre also presented immediate results and mid-term outcome of provisional T-stenting of the side branch in type 2 lesions (lesion proximal and distal to the bifurcation without significant lesion of the side branch), type 3 (lesion of the main branch proximal to the bifurcation) and type 4a (lesion distal to the bifurcation) (slide 12).[45] Among 936 bifurcational lesions consecutively included, 452 (49%) were 'false' and 319 were treated by this approach. The clinical characteristics were similar in each group, and the angiographic success rates were 96, 95, and 100% in type 2, type 3 and type 4a groups, respectively. Seven-month TVR rates (7.5, 5.4, and 16.7%) and MACE rates (11.5, 5.4, and 18.5%) were encouraging, with slightly higher event rates in type 4a lesions ($p<0.05$) compared with type 2 and type 3 lesions.

From a large single-center database of 1149 patients with bifurcational lesions treated between 1996 and 2002, the following predictive factors of TVR were identified: (1) clinical presentation as acute coronary syndrome (OR=6.74); (2) reference diameter ≤ 2.7 mm (OR=2.03); (3) the technique of provisional T-stenting of the SB was a protective factor (OR=0.46) (slide 13).[46]

Drug-eluting stents the Bifurcation Study (slides 14–18).[47] The Bifurcation Study was a five-center randomized trial to assess the feasibility and safety of the treatment of patients with sirolimus-eluting stents at true bifurcational lesions (>50% stenosis in both the main vessel and ostium of the side branch). Two different strategies were used: Group A – elective use of two sirolimus-eluting stents and Group B – the implantation of a single sirolimus-eluting stent in the main vessel with balloon dilatation across the stent struts for the SB. The protocol allowed the investigators to switch to kissing stenting if flow impairment or residual ostial stenosis >50%

developed in the side branch. Twenty-two out of 43 patients randomized to group B crossed over, resulting in implantation of two stents. In-hospital target-vessel failure rate was similar in the two groups (9.5% vs. 9.1%). Angiographic follow-up was performed in 78% of patients. The restenosis rate in the main vessel was 5.7% in group A and 4.8% in group B. The side-branch restenosis rate was less impressive (21.8% vs. 14.2% in groups A and B, respectively). High cross-over rates have made direct comparison of the two groups difficult, but the use of a second drug-eluting stent did not seem to improve the restenosis rate (24.0% in group A and 18.7% in group B). There was focal restenosis at the ostium of the side branch in 14 out of 15 cases. Angiography and/or intravascular ultrasound demonstrated incomplete ostial coverage in two-thirds of the restenosis cases. Target vessel failure rate was 19% in group A and 13.6% in group B.

The most important messages of this study are:

- Compared with historical studies utilizing bare-metal stents,[6,7,10,42,43] a remarkable improvement has been achieved in the treatment of bifurcational lesions when one (main branch) or two stents (main branch and side branch) are implanted
- The side branch appears to be the weak link in the chain in terms of a higher risk of angiographic restenosis (still around 20%) and a slightly higher risk of thrombosis
- When possible, placement of one single stent on the main branch gives a similar result to the placement of two stents
- Suboptimal coverage with struts and drugs at the ostium of the side branch are possible contributing factors to side-branch restenosis

A paper discussing initial experiences with drug-eluting stents for bifurcational lesions in 'real-world' patients was presented at the 2004 ACC meeting by Dr Colombo, Dr Serruys, and Dr Lefevre (slides 19–22). Although there was a difference in stenting technique used (100% crush stenting in Milan, 100% provisional T-stenting in Massy, and a combination of various stenting techniques in Rotterdam – but always with stent placement in both branches) optimal angiographic success and engorging reduction in the incidence of adverse events at follow-up were reported.

CONCLUSIONS

In conclusion, bifurcational stenting demands an appropriate balance between procedural risk and long-term result in achieving an optimal result. The introduction of drug-eluting stents has shown the potential to achieve superb immediate results, which are, according to preliminary reports, maintained at the follow-up. The Sirolimus Bifurcation Study, with all the limitations of being the very first study utilizing a drug-eluting stent, demonstrated almost suppression of restenosis in the main branch. In the side branch, restenosis occurred in about one out of five lesions treated; we cannot dismiss the fact that this restenosis was almost always focal and therefore quite simple in its treatment. We believe that the learning curve with this new device (particularly when implanting two stents) may have contributed to these adverse events. However, there are still several questions unanswered (slide 23). We still have to evaluate the necessity for final kissing balloon inflation when drug-eluting stents are used, and we have to await the results with other stenting techniques, as culottes or V-stenting. The current appropriate application of provisional stenting and refinement of stent techniques when implanting two stents will further improve the results. Finally, the introduction of drug-eluting dedicated stents for different types of bifurcations may further facilitate the conquest of one of the most challenging areas in interventional cardiology.

REFERENCES

1. Pinkerton CA, Slack JD. Complex coronary angioplasty: a technique for dilatation of bifurcation stenoses. Angiology 1985; 36: 543–8
2. Renkin J, Wijns W, Hanet C, et al. Angioplasty of coronary bifurcation stenoses: immediate and long-term results of the protecting branch technique. Cathet Cardiovasc Diagn 1991; 22: 167–73
3. Krams R, Wentzel JJ, Oomen JA, et al. Evaluation of endothelial shear stress and 3D geometry as factors determining the development of atherosclerosis and remodeling in human coronary arteries in vivo. Combining 3D reconstruction from angiography and IVUS (ANGUS) with computational fluid dynamics. Arterioscler Thromb Vasc Biol 1997; 17: 2061–5
4. Feldman CL, Ilegbusi OJ, Hu Z, et al. Determination of in vivo velocity and endothelial shear stress patterns with phasic flow in human coronary arteries: A methodology to predict progression of coronary atherosclerosis. Am Heart J 2002; 143: 931–9
5. Koller P, Safian RD. Bifurcation Stenosis. Birmingham: Physicians Press; 1996
6. Lefevre T, Louvard Y, Morice MC, et al. Stenting of bifurcation lesions: classification, treatments, and results. Catheter Cardiovasc Interv 2000; 49: 274–83
7. Lefevre T, Louvard Y, Morice MC, et al. Stenting of bifurcation lesions: a rational approach. J Interv Cardiol 2001; 14: 573–85
8. Melikian N, Di Mario C. Treatment of bifurcation coronary lesions: a review of current techniques and outcome. J Interv Cardiol 2003; 16: 507–13
9. Louvard Y, Lefevre T, Morice MC. Percutaneous coronary intervention for bifurcation coronary disease. Heart 2004; 90: 713–22
10. Al Suwaidi J, Yeh W, Cohen HA, et al. Immediate and one-year outcome in patients with coronary bifurcation lesions in the modern era (NHLBI dynamic registry). Am J Cardiol 2001; 87: 1139–44
11. Meier B, Gruentzig AR, King SB, 3rd, et al. Risk of side branch occlusion during coronary angioplasty. Am J Cardiol 1984; 53: 10–14
12. Zack PM, Ischinger T. Experience with a technique for coronary angioplasty of bifurcational lesions. Cathet Cardiovasc Diagn 1984; 10: 433–43
13. Pinkerton CA, Slack JD, Van Tassel JW, Orr CM. Angioplasty for dilatation of complex coronary artery bifurcation stenoses. Am J Cardiol 1985; 55: 1626–8
14. George BS, Myler RK, Stertzer SH, et al. Balloon angioplasty of coronary bifurcation lesions: the kissing balloon technique. Cathet Cardiovasc Diagn 1986; 12: 124–38

15. Oesterle SN, McAuley BJ, Buchbinder M, Simpson JB. Angioplasty at coronary bifurcations: single-guide, two-wire technique. Cathet Cardiovasc Diagn 1986; 12: 57–63

16. Vallbracht C, Kober G, Kaltenbach M. Double long-wire technique for percutaneous transluminal coronary angioplasty for narrowings at major bifurcations. Am J Cardiol 1987; 60: 907–9

17. Fischman DL, Savage MP, Leon MB, et al. Fate of lesion-related side branches after coronary artery stenting. J Am Coll Cardiol 1993; 22: 1641–6

18. Vetrovec GW, Cowley MJ, Wolfgang TC, Ducey KC. Effects of percutaneous transluminal coronary angioplasty on lesion-associated branches. Am Heart J 1985; 109: 921–5

19. Boxt LM, Meyerovitz MF, Taus RH, et al. Side branch occlusion complicating percutaneous transluminal coronary angioplasty. Radiology 1986; 161: 681–3

20. Dardas PS, Tsikaderis DD, Mezilis NE, Styliadis G. A technique for type 4a coronary bifurcation lesions: initial results and 6-month clinical evaluation. J Invasive Cardiol 2003; 15: 180–3

21. Adelman AG, Cohen EA, Kimball BP, et al. A comparison of directional atherectomy with balloon angioplasty for lesions of the left anterior descending coronary artery. N Engl J Med 1993; 329: 228–33

22. Boehrer JD, Ellis SG, Pieper K, et al. Directional atherectomy versus balloon angioplasty for coronary ostial and nonostial left anterior descending coronary artery lesions: results from a randomized multicenter trial. The CAVEAT-I investigators. Coronary Angioplasty Versus Excisional Atherectomy Trial. J Am Coll Cardiol 1995; 25: 1380–6

23. Karvouni E, Di Mario C, Nishida T, et al. Directional atherectomy prior to stenting in bifurcation lesions: a matched comparison study with stenting alone. Catheter Cardiovasc Interv 2001; 53: 12–20

24. Heintzen MP, Aktug O, Michel CJ. Debulking prior to stenting – a worthwhile effort? Z Kardiol 2002; 91 Suppl 3: 72–6

25. Serruys PW, de Jaegere P, Kiemeneij F, et al. A comparison of balloon-expandable-stent implantation with balloon angioplasty in patients with coronary artery disease. Benestent Study Group. N Engl J Med 1994; 331: 489–95

26. Fischman DL, Leon MB, Baim DS, et al. A randomized comparison of coronary-stent placement and balloon angioplasty in the treatment of coronary artery disease. Stent Restenosis Study Investigators. N Engl J Med 1994; 331: 496–501

27. Aliabadi D, Tilli FV, Bowers TR, et al. Incidence and angiographic predictors of side branch occlusion following high-pressure intracoronary stenting. Am J Cardiol 1997; 80: 994–7

28. Pan M, Medina A, Suarez de Lezo J, et al. Follow-up patency of side branches covered by intracoronary Palmaz–Schatz stent. Am Heart J 1995; 129: 436–40

29. Arora RR, Raymond RE, Dimas AP, et al. Side branch occlusion during coronary angioplasty: incidence, angiographic characteristics, and outcome. Cathet Cardiovasc Diagn 1989; 18: 210–12

30. Bhargava B, Waksman R, Lansky AJ, et al. Clinical outcomes of compromised side branch (stent jail) after coronary stenting with the NIR stent. Catheter Cardiovasc Interv 2001; 54: 295–300

31. Colombo A, Gaglione A, Nakamura S, Finci L. 'Kissing' stents for bifurcational coronary lesion. Cathet Cardiovasc Diagn 1993; 30: 327–30

32. Nakamura S, Hall P, Maiello L, Colombo A. Techniques for Palmaz–Schatz stent deployment in lesions with a large side branch. Cathet Cardiovasc Diagn 1995; 34: 353–61

33. Carrie D, Karouny E, Chouairi S, Puel J. 'T'-shaped stent placement: a technique for the treatment of dissected bifurcation lesions. Cathet Cardiovasc Diagn 1996; 37: 311–13

34. Fort S, Lazzam C, Schwartz L. Coronary 'Y' stenting: a technique for angioplasty of bifurcation stenoses. Can J Cardiol 1996; 12: 678–82

35. Schampaert E, Fort S, Adelman AG, Schwartz L. The V-stent: a novel technique for coronary bifurcation stenting. Cathet Cardiovasc Diagn 1996; 39: 320–6

36. Khoja A, Ozbek C, Bay W, Heisel A. Trouser-like stenting: a new technique for bifurcation lesions. Cathet Cardiovasc Diagn 1997; 41: 192–6; discussion 197–9

37. Di Mario C, Colombo A. Trousers-stents: How to choose the right size and shape? Cathet Cardiovasc Diagn 1997; 41: 197–9

38. Chevalier B, Glatt B, Royer T, Guyon P. Placement of coronary stents in bifurcation lesions by the 'culotte' technique. Am J Cardiol 1998; 82: 943–9

39. Kobayashi Y, Colombo A, Akiyama T, et al. Modified 'T' stenting: a technique for kissing stents in bifurcational coronary lesion. Cathet Cardiovasc Diagn 1998; 43: 323–6

40. Kobayashi Y, Colombo A, Adamian M, et al. The skirt technique: A stenting technique to treat a lesion immediately proximal to the bifurcation (pseudobifurcation). Catheter Cardiovasc Interv 2000; 51: 347–51

41. Colombo A, Stankovic G, Orlic D, et al. Modified T-stenting technique with crush for bifurcation lesions: immediate results and 30-day outcome. Catheter Cardiovasc Interv 2003; 60: 145–51

42. Yamashita T, Nishida T, Adamian MG, et al. Bifurcation lesions: two stents versus one stent – immediate and follow-up results. J Am Coll Cardiol 2000; 35: 1145–51

43. Al Suwaidi J, Berger PB, Rihal CS, et al. Immediate and long-term outcome of intracoronary stent implantation for true bifurcation lesions. J Am Coll Cardiol 2000; 35: 929–36

44. Lefevre T, Louvard Y, Morice MC, et al. Evaluation of different approaches to stenting true bifurcation lesions (abstract). Eur Heart J 2002; 4: 2682

45. Lefevre T, Louvard Y, Morice MC, et al. Treatment of 'false bifurcation lesions' with coronary stenting (abstract). Eur Heart J 2002; 4: 2050

46. Lefevre T, Sengottuvel G, Kokis A, et al. Predictors of target vessel revascularization after stenting coronary bifurcation lesions: insights from a large prospective single-center database (abstract). J Am Coll Cardiol 2004; 43 (Suppl A): 1081–150

47. Colombo A, Moses JW, Morice MC, et al. Randomized study to evaluate sirolimus-eluting stents implanted at coronary bifurcation lesions. Circulation 2004; 109: 1244–9

Case examples

1. Stenting the main branch and dilating the side branch (provisional stenting)

Case # 11723/03

This case (**slides 1–4** (*frames 1–10*)) illustrates a long diseased area in the proximal and mid-left anterior descending (LAD) with a lesion in the diagonal branch. The diagonal branch is diseased, and one standard approach could be to use a classic crushing technique. The operator in this case preferred to use a provisional approach, planning to stent the LAD and dilate the diagonal without a stent. *Frames 3* and *4* show our standard approach when dealing with an ostial diagonal lesion. The vessel is treated with a 6-mm-long cutting balloon. *Frame 5* shows the results which appear acceptable at the level of the diagonal branch. *Frames 6* and *7* show deployment of a Taxus stent (Boston Scientific) at the level of the LAD. The kissing inflation, following recrossing into the diagonal, is shown in *frame 9* and the final result in *frame 10*.

Message This case shows that frequently the side branch can be treated only with balloon dilatation and that stenting should be reserved primarily for the main branch. Of course, this good result is not always a guarantee and, if needed, the next step would have been a reverse crushing with a stent protruding from the diagonal into the LAD.

2. The classical 'crush' technique

Case # 11162/02

This is a typical example (**slides 1–4** (*frames 1–8*); and **slides 5–9**) for which we recommend double stent implantation and we avoid provisional stenting. The reasons for this decision are the following:

(1) There is involvement of both branches, left anterior descending (LAD) and diagonal.
(2) Both branches are large in size and are important as regards the territory of distribution.

(3) The diagonal branch has a lesion immediately after the bifurcation. For this task, the use of a long stent will take care not only of the bifurcational lesion, but also of the distal lesion. The decision to use two stents becomes almost cost-effective.

The approach we use in this situation, following wiring of both branches, is to fully pre-dilate the diagonal branch and LAD. It has been our practice to use the cutting balloon to pre-dilate, particularly the ostium of the side branch. Like in most of the ostial lesions, preparation of the lesion with a cutting balloon is one of the best approaches to completely open the lesion and to allow full stent expansion at the ostium of the diagonal with better contact of the stent struts and the wall. This fact may be of particular value when implanting a drug-eluting stent.

Following this pre-dilatation, which it is important to carry out using the appropriate size of cutting balloon (avoiding undersizing this device), the stents are implanted with the usual crushing technique. *Frame 4* illustrates the inflation first of the long stent in the diagonal, which covers the ostial lesion as well as the tandem lesion in the diagonal. The stent in the LAD is in place with a proximal mark, more proximally than the mark in the diagonal branch. Following deployment of the stent in the diagonal, the stent in the LAD is inflated after having removed balloon and wires from the diagonal branch. The final result, following kissing inflation, is demonstrated in two projections in *frames 5* and *6*. It is evident how well expanded the stent is at the ostium of the diagonal, most probably due not only to the kissing inflation, but also to appropriate pre-dilatation of the ostium of this branch. In *frames 7* and *8*, we see the 10-month angiographic follow-up in two projections. We are showing this full example because we believe that this approach is the optimal strategy for the crush technique following all the phases of evolution of this approach for bifurcations.

The only element that may be missing from this case is IVUS evaluation of the appropriate size of the side branch. We believe that frequently it is necessary to perform IVUS, particularly at the level of the side branch, in order not to undersize the cutting balloon that is used to pre-dilate the diagonal branch.

Tips Regarding cutting-balloon sizing and the possible risk of perforation, it is important to undersize the cutting balloon ≥ 0.5 mm, from the IVUS measurements of media to media, if the origin of the diagonal is close to 90°. This condition, particularly if the lesion is fibrotic or calcific, may increase the risk of perforation due to the rigid blades of the cutting balloon.

To re-cross into the diagonal branch, we try first the same wire we used originally, then the second choice is a Pilot 50 or 150 (Guidant).

If a new 1.5-mm balloon does not cross into the diagonal, we may consider rewiring, or, in other circumstances, we may use the Ace balloon (balloon with a fixed-wire system, from Boston Scientific).

3. 'Double crush' technique

Case # HSR 32290

This case (**slides 1–5** (*frames 1–11*)) illustrates a complex approach to a trifurcational lesion with the technique of double crushing. In this case, the lesion involves the distal part of the left main with involvement of the left anterior descending, ramus, and the circumflex. *Frames 1* and *2* illustrate the baseline anatomy. Following balloon pre-dilatation as shown in *frame 3* (today optimally performed with a cutting balloon while, at that time, it was done with regular balloon), the stents are positioned. In this particular case, we consider the final stent as the one in the left anterior descending; the intermediate is the one in the circumflex and the first stent is the one in the ramus. The first stent is the one that has the marker positioned most distally and is the one that is deployed first (*frame 4*). Then the balloon and the wire are removed from the ramus and the second stent, which is the one in the circumflex, is deployed (*frame 6*). Following deployment of this stent and removal of the guidewire and balloon from the circumflex, the left anterior descending stent is deployed (*frame 7*). The final step necessitates rewiring the circumflex and the ramus. Sometimes one of the two branches is rewired with a fixed-wire balloon like the Ace balloon and kissing inflation is performed with three balloons. The final result is shown in *frames 8* and *9*. In this patient, the 6-months angiographic follow-up has been reasonably gratifying without any re-narrowing as shown in *frames 10* and *11*. The main advantage of this approach, particularly in the distal left main lesion, is that immediate patency is assured in all three branches, and the only complex task is to rewire to perform kissing inflation. An alternative approach would have been to utilize a classic crush with the LAD and the circumflex and a provisional stent of the ramus, or even a more simple V-technique with stenting of the circumflex and the LAD and, again, provisional stenting of the ramus branch. As is true in many circumstances, these bifurcational lesions can usually be treated in more than one fashion, and the decision is sometimes dependent on the level of confidence that each operator has with a certain technique and his results at follow-up.

Tip   At least a 9-Fr guiding catheter is needed to allow simultaneous placement of three stents.

4. Intravascular ultrasound (IVUS) documentation of the result following the crush stenting technique

Case # 11591/03

This example (**slides 1–3** (*frames 1–11*)) shows a crush technique with IVUS documentation of the results. A baseline lesion is shown in *frame 1*. It is important to state first that, in this case, an alternative approach to the crush technique would have been provisional stenting of the side branch, most probably of the posterior descending. In this case, the operator adopted to stent both branches.

Frames 2 and *3* show that there is disease localized primarily in the distal right coronary artery with some involvement of the ostium of the postero-lateral branch at the IVUS evaluation. Following pre-dilatation, two Taxus stents are deployed with the classic crushing technique, regarding the posterior descending as the main branch. For that reason, the first stent to be implanted and inflated is the stent in the postero-lateral branch (*frame 5*).

The next step is to inflate the stent into the distal right coronary towards the posterior descending. *Frame 7* shows the final kissing. The final result, with the corresponding IVUS image, is seen in *frames 8* and *9*. It is pleasing to realize that, following optimal kissing, an IVUS catheter can be advanced towards the posterior descending and towards the postero-lateral branches. *Frames 10* and *11* show the result at these two sites, with optimal opening of the stent struts towards both branches.

The availability of an open-cell stent design is most probably an optimal tool, particularly when dealing with these large branches which may require a final diameter at their ostium larger than 3 mm.

5. 'Reverse' crush due to provisional stent strategy

Case # 11497/03

This is an example (**slides 1–9** (*frames 1–14, runs 1–5*); and **slides 10–15**) of an ostial lesion of the left anterior descending, with some distal disease in the left main coronary artery. The distal left main trifurcates, with the large intermediate branch and the smaller circumflex branch (*frames 1–3*). It is important to point out that both these two branches are relatively free of disease, and this is the reason why the operator first selected to use only one stent positioned from the distal left main towards the LAD. *Frame 4* shows the deployment of a single 3.5 × 18-mm-long Cypher stent (Cordis). *Frame 5* shows the initial result following stent deployment. It is relatively clear that the ostium of the intermediate branch is slightly compromised. Keeping with the original plan to stent only the LAD, the operator first tried side-branch dilatation towards the intermediate and then kissing. Both these steps are shown in the two panels, *frames 7* and *8*. *Frame 9* and (*run 4*) show the result following kissing. Despite maintained patency of the intermediate and of the circumflex, the ostium of the intermediate branch did not appear satisfactory. For this reason, a stent needed to be implanted at this level.

Owing to the fact that a stent is already in place in the LAD, we needed to utilize the 'reverse crush' technique. This technique is used with a stand-by balloon in the left anterior descending, which will be used to crush the protruding part of the stent from the intermediate branch into the LAD. *Frame 10* shows stent deployment into the intermediate. The stent is protruding into the LAD, and a 3.5-mm balloon is parked in the left anterior descending ready to be inflated following stent deployment. *Frame 11* shows that wire and balloon have been removed from the intermediate branch, and now the balloon in the LAD is crushing the protruding part of the stent from the intermediate branch into the LAD. The next step is to recross into the intermediate branch and perform kissing inflation (*frames 12 and 13*). The final result is shown in *frame 14*. In this case, thanks to the 90° origin of the circumflex, it does not seem important or necessary to perform any additional inflation into the circumflex. It is evident that an optimal result is present at the ostium of the intermediate branch as well as of the LAD.

Message   The most important message of this case is the initial consideration not to stent a side branch if this branch is not diseased. The other message is that in case, following stent deployment into the main branch and following kissing inflation, there is the need to stent the ostium of the other branch, this goal can be accomplished utilizing reverse crush. The only limitation of reverse crush is that occasionally there may be difficulties in advancing the second stent across the struts of the first stent into the side branch. If the side branch is severely angulated, it may be wise to use a classic crush technique in order to minimize the risk of performing reverse crush should the result following left main stenting be considered inadequate.

Another common approach to deal with these conditions is to perform T-stenting at the origin of the side branch. Again, the major limitation that we see with T-stenting is that the stent on the side branch may not fully cover the ostium of this branch, and drug delivery may not be performed optimally at this level. Reverse crush attempts to address this problem.

6. The 'inverse' crush technique

Case # 11728/03

This example (**slides 1–3** (*frames 1–8*); and **slides 4–8**) illustrates a variation of the crush technique called 'inverse' crush (different from 'reverse' crush). The disease is mainly confined at the ostium of the diagonal branch. Owing to the fact that the origin of the diagonal branch is relatively angulated, a single stent positioned at the ostium of the diagonal branch would compromise the left anterior descending, which also appears relatively diseased at this level. For this reason, we decided to stent both branches. We could have utilized the standard crush technique; the reason why we are demonstrating the use of inverse crush is to show an approach that makes crossing for final kissing relatively easy.

One limitation of the inverse crush technique is that this approach needs to be used with a stent for which the cells can be fully opened, if necessary at almost any diameter. This need is due to the fact that the cell of the stent positioned into the diagonal branch has to be opened towards the LAD. *Frames 1* and *2* illustrate the baseline lesion characteristics. In **slide 2**, we see four frames with the various steps of this inverse crush technique. *Frame 3* shows pre-dilatation towards the diagonal branch. *Frame 4* shows both stents in place, a long stent in the diagonal and a shorter stent in the LAD, protruding proximal to the bifurcation but distally to the stent into the diagonal branch. *Frame 5* shows that the first stent to be inflated is the LAD stent. Following this step and following removal of the balloon and of the wire from the LAD, the stent in the diagonal branch is inflated (*frame 6*). The procedure is completed with final kissing balloon inflation (**slide 3** (*frame 7*)). It is easier to recross the stent towards the LAD which follows a less angulated pathway. This is one of the reasons why the operator may prefer the inverse crush approach.

As mentioned earlier, the limitation of this technique is the fact that the stent towards the diagonal branch needs to be opened towards the LAD (like culottes), and the struts of this stent need to allow this maximum opening, which sometimes needs to reach 3.5 mm in diameter. In order to perform this technique, we must use an open-cell stent. A closed-cell stent like the Cypher is not suitable for the inverse crush technique.

The main advantage of this technique, as mentioned earlier, is the fact that the recrossing for final kissing may be easier because it is performed towards the least angulated branch.

7. The T-stenting technique

Case # 10706/02

This is an example (**slides 1–3** (*frames 1–7*; and **slides 4–8**)) of a bifurcational lesion in which the ostium of the diagonal branch is relatively preserved. The baseline images show this fact in *frames 1* and 2. For reasons mentioned earlier, the operator decides to stent only the LAD. *Frames 3* and *4* show positioning of the stent and the result following stent placement in the left anterior descending. Owing to inadequate results at the ostium of the diagonal branch, shown in *frame 4*, the operator decides to stent the ostium of the diagonal branch. *Frames 5* and *6* show this procedure performed with a classic T-stenting technique. T-stenting, compared with the crush technique, does not consider making the stent of the diagonal protrude into the LAD. As shown in *frame 6*, both balloons are inflated in a kissing way without removing the wire and recrossing into the diagonal. This maneuver is possible because the stents are just close to each other and not overlapping. *Frame 7* shows the final result.

The T-stenting technique appears relatively easy to perform, the only limitation being that the stent into the side branch may be difficult to negotiate into that branch. The other limitation of this technique is the fact that we can never be completely certain that the ostium of the diagonal branch will be fully covered with struts and that drug delivery will be completely accomplished at this level.

8. The V-stenting technique

Case # 10916/02

This case is illustrated by **slides 1–4** (*frames 1–10*) and **slides 5–8**. Two baseline frames (*frames 1* and *2*) demonstrate a typical distal lesion of the left main coronary artery with two large branches, LAD and circumflex. A common approach when dealing with these lesions would be to debulk the distal left main, at least towards the LAD. In this case, we chose a simpler and more straightforward approach by utilizing a V-stenting technique. V-stenting was used owing to the fact that the disease was mainly at the level of the very distal left main, and the angle of the two branches was very favorable for a V-technique. *Frames 3* and *4* show stent deployment at the level of the two vessels. It is worth mentioning that the stents utilized were 3-mm Cypher stents (most probably because at that time a 3.5-mm stent was not yet available). Today, we would use a seven-cell 3.5-mm Cypher stent. Subsequently, these stents were then post-dilated (*frame 6*) with a 4-mm balloon. This last step, even if appropriate in order to obtain full stent apposition and maximal lumen diameter, may be questionable, particularly when dealing with a six-cell Cypher stent. Again the use of the 3.5-mm seven-cell Cypher stent would have been more appropriate. The final result is shown in *frames 7* and *8*, which demonstrate optimal patency of both branches.

Despite the lack of debulking and the need to perform over-dilatation of the two stents, the follow-up results demonstrate an absence of restenosis with just a modest re-narrowing at the ostium of the circumflex (*frame 10*) which does not appear angiographically critical. By looking carefully at *frame 6*, which shows the post-dilatation image following dilatation with a 4-mm diameter balloon, it is evident that the mid-portion of the balloon in the circumflex does not appear fully expanded. Perhaps the best compromise in this specific lesion would have been to pre-dilate post-branches with an appropriately sized cutting balloon. We are increasingly inclined to use this device fairly liberally, particularly when dealing with ostial or bifurcational lesions.

Message   The V-technique is certainly the easiest, the safest, and the most predictable technique for dealing with bifurcational lesions. We suggest that this technique should be used in distal left main lesions when the left main trunk is short and free of disease. The fact that the wires are always left in place makes this technique very safe. The main limitation of the V-technique is that if a stent needs to be implanted more proximally, the direction of this stent will necessarily take the one of the main branch, or whatever the operator decides following removal of one wire from the other branch. For this reason, we prefer to use the V-technique only in very proximal lesions, like the left main, or in situations in which there is no disease proximal to the bifurcation and we are fairly certain that an additional stent will not be required.

9. Proximal stenting following V-stenting

Case # 11998/04

This case (**slide 1–8** (*frames 1–18*)) illustrates a rare but important issue: a lesion which needs to be treated following an approach with V-stenting in a bifurcational lesion. *Frames 1* and *2* show the bifurcational lesion at the origin of very angulated obtuse marginal branch. This vessel was entered with some difficulties utilizing a Whisper wire (Guidant). After pre-dilatation, the distal lesion was treated with a 33-mm Cypher stent, as shown in *frame 3*. Then, more aggressive pre-dilatation of the obtuse marginal branch was performed (*frame 4*). At this point, two Taxus stents (*frame 5*) were deployed (*frame 6*) with the V-stent approach. The final result is shown in *frame 7*. Now we face the issue of stenting the more proximal lesion without compromising the V-stent result at the bifurcation site. One approach, which is slightly complex, is to utilize the 'skirt technique'. As demonstrated in *frame 8*, a Taxus stent is disassembled and remounted on a double-balloon system. The two balloons, held together by the stent, are advanced individually in each of the two branches. The balloons are kept together by the stent and, finally, they will allow the stent to open in the appropriate two directions. *Frame 9* demonstrates the deployment of the stent with the guide-wires in each of the two branches. The final result is presented in *frames 10* and *11*.

The lesion in the LAD, presented in *frames 12* and *13*, shows a different approach which we utilized to solve the problem of proximal stenting following V-stenting. The lesion was treated with the implantation of two Taxus stents with a V-technique as shown in *frames 14* and *15*. The final result was satisfactory at the level of the bifurcation, but there is a dissection in the proximal segment as shown in *frame 16*. At this point, instead of utilizing the skirt approach, the operator preferred a more simple approach, which is the conversion of V into crush. A Taxus stent is advanced into the LAD to crush the protruding diagonal stent. The final result following kissing inflation is presented in *frame 18*.

Again, these two examples show a rare, but important, problem of proximal stenting following the V-stenting technique.

10. 'Culottes' stenting technique

Case # 11470/03

This case (**slides 1–5** (*frames 1–12*)) concerns a typical lesion at the bifurcation of the unprotected left main. This lesion was treated utilizing a standard culottes technique, preceded by debulking. *Frames 1* and *2*, besides showing the baseline lesion, show the presence of elective intraaortic balloon pump. We believe that this extra step will guarantee maximal protection during the procedure. This requirement is particularly necessary when performing a complex approach such as culottes stenting, preceded by atherectomy. Both lesions are first wired, as shown in *frame 3*, and then directional atherectomy with the Flexicut (Guidant) is performed towards the LAD. In this case, atherectomy was not so successful because there was a distal sub-occlusive dissection seen at *frame 5*. Immediately following atherectomy, a Taxus stent is deployed towards the LAD. It is worth mentioning that, at this critical moment, the presence of a balloon pump is of great help and security. Following stent deployment, usually not at high pressure, but around 10 atm, it is evident that the origin of the circumflex is compromised. The circumflex is rewired, and balloon dilatation is performed at this level. Following this step, another Taxus stent is advanced towards the circumflex (*frame 9*). This advancement of the stent into the circumflex is a critical element of the culottes technique, which accomplishes overlap of the two stents in the proximal segment of the bifurcation, with final opening of the struts towards each side branch. Owing to the fact that the proximal left main is a relatively large vessel, double struts and double drug medication at this level appear to be the advantage of this approach.

Frame 10 shows kissing inflation, which is performed following the rewiring towards the LAD. Kissing inflation is carried out in order to open both struts towards each vessel. The reason why the operator decided to utilize the Taxus stent rather than the Cypher stent is related to the choice of the culotte technique. When utilizing this technique, particulary if the diameters of the vessels are >3 mm, it is essential to use a stent with an open-cell design, which allows opening all the cells to a diameter >3 mm when necessary. A limitation of a stent with a closed-cell design, like the Cypher stent, is that the cell struts will open only to a maximum diameter of 3 mm. For this reason, we prefer not to use the Cypher when we decide to perform the culottes technique. *Frames 11* and *12* show the final result following kissing inflation.

Message   The culottes technique is not easy and may be fairly time consuming. In an unprotected situation like left main stenting, it should ideally be used with extreme caution, owing to the fact that the operator needs to temporarily lose access from one branch (usually the most important branch, because the first stent needs to be positioned in the most angulated branch; this step was not done in such a way in the case just described owing to the fact that there was an initial dissection in the LAD, and this vessel needed immediate treatment). Despite these limitations, the culottes technique is the approach which gives the best coverage of the ostium of both branches and which may optimize drug delivery.

11. Creating a 'funnel' or 'pseudobifurcation' technique

Case # 34101HSR

This case (slides 1–5 (*frames 1–9* and *runs 1, 2*)) shows a particular technique, which we can define as work in progress, because it requires some modification of the device. *Frames 1* and *2* show a baseline lesion in the proximal LAD which is mainly located at the proximal part of a bifurcation with the diagonal branch. The most standard approach in this situation would be to place one stent in the LAD, covering the ostium of the diagonal branch, and then to perform kissing balloon inflation if necessary towards the diagonal branch. A more sophisticated, and somehow more elegant, approach is to wire both branches and then deploy a stent mounted on two balloons. These two balloons will open the stent like a skirt towards the diagonal branch and towards the LAD. *Frame 5* shows a Taxus stent which has been partially expanded in order to allow another Maverick balloon (Boston Scientific) to be crimped inside the stent. This construction allows the advancement of two balloons over two wires, with one stent keeping the two balloons together. *Frame 4* shows that the stent stops at the carina following the resistance encountered by the distal part of the stent against the bifurcation. *Run 1* shows optimal positioning of the stent which is implanted with inflation of both balloons. *Frame 6* shows an interesting tip: partial retrieval of the wire from the diagonal branch in order to allow the most floppy part of the wire to be in contact with the tip of the balloon and facilitate its deflection towards the diagonal branch. The final result is shown in *Frames 7* and *8*, with optimal opening of the stent towards both branches. This angiographic result is confirmed in the IVUS pull back, which shows a distal wide opening of the stent towards the LAD and towards the diagonal branch.

We believe that this technique is appropriate for bifurcational lesions in which the disease is confined in the proximal part of the bifurcation. Unfortunately, no company supplies a stent pre-mounted on two balloons. In order to use this approach, the operator needs to assemble two devices.

12. A bifurcational lesion: stenting from the main to the side branch

Case # 36474HSR

This case (**slides 1–4** (*frames 1–10*)) illustrates what we call a practical and economical approach to bifurcational lesions. The baseline angiogram depicted in *Frames 1* and *2* shows the proximal ostial lesion of the left anterior descending and a lesion of the first diagonal branch. The approach taken in this case was to use a long stent going from the ostium of the LAD into the diagonal branch and to perform provisionally angioplasty on the mid-LAD post-bifurcation. *Frames 3* and *4* show predilatation of the diagonal branch then, *frames 5* and *6* show deployment of a Taxus 2.5 × 32-mm stent going from the ostium of the LAD into the diagonal. This long stent was able to cover both lesions. It is important to remember that the 2.5-mm stent is the same as the one mounted on 3.0 and 3.5-mm balloons and therefore can be easily dilated to these larger diameters. *Frames 7* and *8* show kissing inflation and then a post-dilatation of the left anterior descending. The final result is shown in *Frames 9* and *10*.

Message   The message of this case is that a bifurcational lesion without involvement of the left anterior descending or the side branch can be treated with one stent, and the unusual aspect of this case is that, for practical reasons, the side branch was considered almost to be the main branch.

13. Measurement of fractional flow reserve (FFR) in a restenotic ostial lesion

Case # 11005/02

This case (**slides 1–4** (*frames 1–8*)) illustrates the value of functional lesion evalua-tion. *Frames 1* and *2* show a lesion in the left anterior descending at the bifurcation with a relatively medium-sized diagonal branch. It is important to notice that the diagonal branch does not appear to be diseased, but the two branches originate with a very narrow angle. This narrow angle increases the risk of compromising the diag-onal branch when a stent is implanted in the left anterior descending. One traditional approach would be to revaluate following stent implantation in the LAD and following kissing balloon inflation towards the diagonal. If the result did not appear adequate, a reverse crush technique could be performed at that time. In this specific case, the operator decided to perform elective double stent implantation with the crush technique. This is demonstrated in *frame 3*, with a final result shown in *frame 4*. The follow-up result at 7 months, with a patient totally asymptomatic, shows good patency of the stent towards the LAD and apparent good patency of the stent in the diagonal branch in the cranial RAO projection (*frame 5*). A slightly different angulation shows that the ostium of the diagonal branch appears focally narrowed. *Frame 7*, with magnification, clearly shows this focal narrowing. An evaluation of this lesion with the pressure-wire confirmed that this focal narrowing was not functionally significant, giving a fractional flow reserve of 0.91 following intracoronary administration of adenosine. It is worth mentioning that, despite the unsuccessful crossing of the IVUS catheter, this lesion proved not to be critical. No events occurred at follow-up, which now extends over 1 year. The important message of this specific case is that many of those very focal narrowings, despite being critical from the angiographic point of view, may not have a clinical impact even following careful search for any demonstrable ischemia.

Message   Many ostial angiographically critical lesions, particularly if very focal, may not be associated with any demonstrable ischemia. If the patient is asymp-tomatic, consider nonintervention, or evaluate the lesion with a pressure gradient fol-lowing adenosine administration. Some restenotic lesions, such as the one presented here, may not be evaluated by IVUS owing to the presence of a stent in the main branch and due to the angle of origin of the side branch.

14. V-stenting for trifurcation lesion

Case # 119591

This case is illustrated by **slides 1–4** (*frames 1–11*). Use of a V-technique is particularly useful in bifurcations with minimal or no proximal disease, or for bifurcations which are located at the ostium of the LAD and of the circumflex, when the left main does not need to be stented. If a lesion involves a trifurcation, the advantages of a V-technique are even more evident. *Frame 1* displays a large inter-mediate branch as a part of a trifurcation with the LAD and circumflex. The left main is large, as shown in *frame 2*, and free of disease. Following wiring of the three branches and after treatment of a more distal lesion in the LAD with Cypher stents, the LAD, intermediate, and circumflex lesions are treated. The guiding catheter uti-lized is at least a 9-Fr catheter, able to accommodate three stents simultaneously. The lesions are pre-dilated, and with three wires in place, three stents are positioned in a W-technique. Each stent is individually inflated in order to avoid slippage. Finally, a simultaneous kissing balloon inflation is performed as shown in *frame 9*. The final result is presented in *frames 10* and *11*. The advantages of this technique are obvious and are due to the absence of recrossing the stents and the maintenance of access to each branch during the entire procedure.

15. V-stenting for trifurcation lesion

Case # 11961

This is another example (**slides 1–6** (*frames 1–17*)) of a trifurcation involving the distal left main treated with a V-technique. What is striking in this case is the initial small size of the intermediate branch, which the operator may dismiss as the less important vessel. The fact that the vessel extends almost to the apex, as shown in *frame 1*, should alert the operator to the reality that this is not a secondary artery.

First the LAD lesions are treated as shown in *frames 2, 3*, and *4*, and then the intermediate branch is pre-dilated with the standard balloon and cutting balloon as shown in *frames 6* and *7*.

Following placement of the stent in the mid-part of the intermediate branch, it is clear that this branch is much more than a secondary ramus. Now the need to treat the ostial of these three arteries becomes evident in the examination of *frame 10*. The approach selected is again V-stenting, which appears to be the easiest and the most effective technique for covering the three branches without the need to stent the left main. Notice the presence of a balloon pump in the aorta as shown in *frame 11*. This help is very important, because the positioning of the three stents in the left main may obstruct the flow in the three arteries and may not achieve enough time for the operator to be precise in the alignment of the three stents in the proper position. A 9-Fr guide-catheter is used. The three stents are first deployed individually as shown in *frames 11–13*, and then a final kissing balloon inflation is performed (*frame 14*). *Frames 15–17* show the final result in three projections.

Didactic crushing cases

In order to make crush stenting technique more comprehensive and easier to perform we provide the following case examples with the corresponding schematic drawings.

STANDARD CRUSHING (CASE # 11645/04) (SLIDES 1–9)

Crushing technique

(1) Wire branches and pre-dilate
(2) Both stents in place: main-branch stent more proximal
(3) Deploy the side-branch stent
(4) Deploy main-branch stent following removal balloon and wire from side branch
(5) Rewire the side branch and perform high-pressure dilatation
(6) Kissing at medium pressure

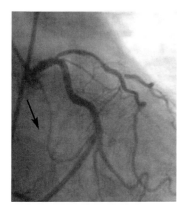
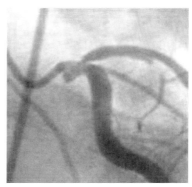

Baseline

Figure 1   Crush technique

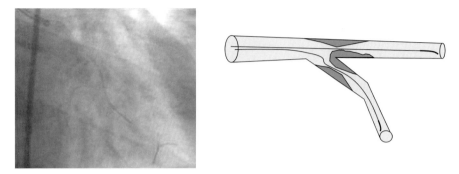

Figure 2   Crush technique. Step 1: Wire both branches and pre-dilate both

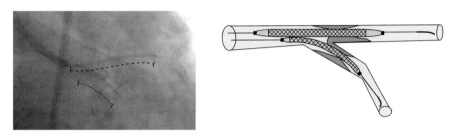

Figure 3   Crush technique. Step 2: Both stents in place. Main branch stent positioned more proximal

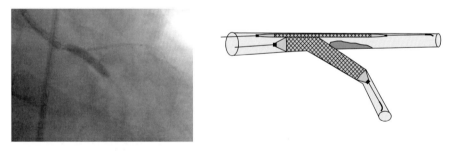

Figure 4   Crush technique. Step 3: Deploy the side-branch stent

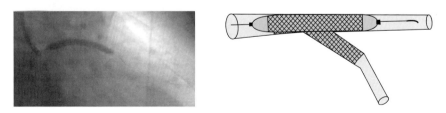

Figure 5   Crush technique. Step 4: Remove balloon and wire from side branch and deploy main-branch stent

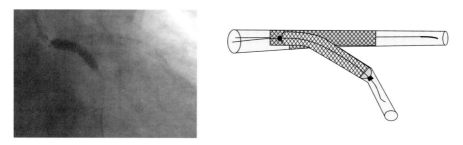

Figure 6 Crush technique. Step 5: Rewire the side branch and perform high pressure dilatation

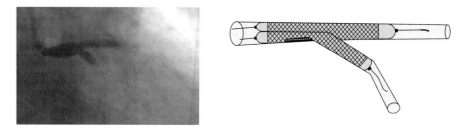

Figure 7 Crush technique. Step 6: Kissing inflation at medium pressure

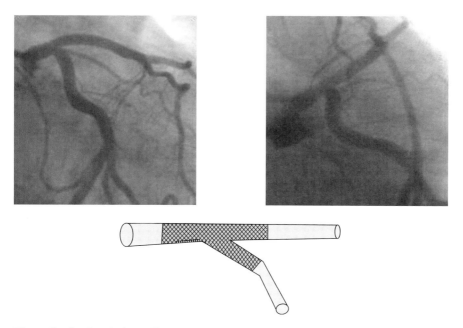

Figure 8 Crush technique. Final result

INVERSE CRUSHING TECHNIQUE (CASE # 11989/043) (SLIDES 1–9)

(1) Wire branches and pre-dilate
(2) Both stents in place: side-branch stent more proximal
(3) Deploy main-branch stent and remove balloon and wire
(4) Deploy the side-branch stent and crush part of the main-branch stent
(5) Rewire the main branch and perform high-pressure dilatation
(6) Kissing at medium pressure

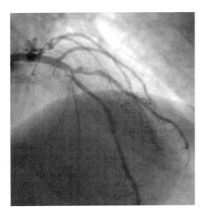 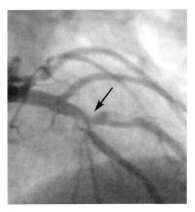

Baseline

Figure 1   Inverse crushing technique

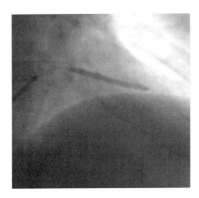 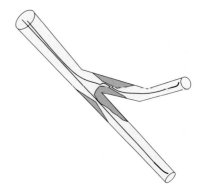

Figure 2   Inverse crushing technique. Step 1: Wire both branches and pre-dilate both

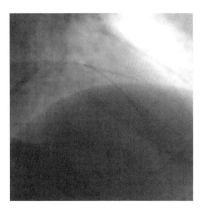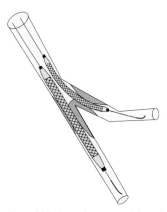

Figure 3 Inverse crushing technique. Step 2: Both stents in place. Side-branch stent positioned more proximal

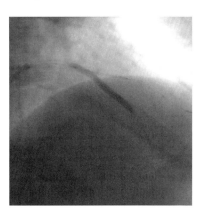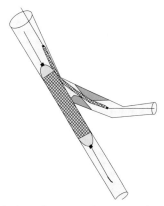

Figure 4 Inverse crushing technique. Step 3: Deploy main-branch stent and remove wire and balloon

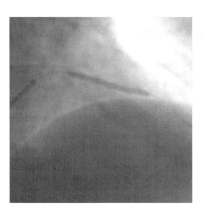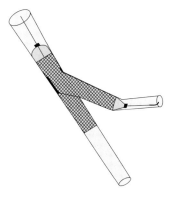

Figure 5 Inverse crushing technique. Step 4: Deploy the side-branch stent and crush part of the main-branch stent

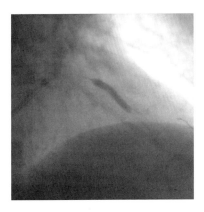
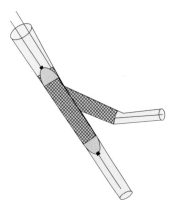

Figure 6 Inverse crushing technique. Step 5: Rewire the main branch and perform high-pressure dilatation

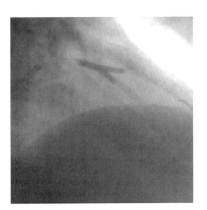
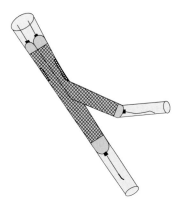

Figure 7 Inverse crushing technique. Step 6: Kissing at medium pressure

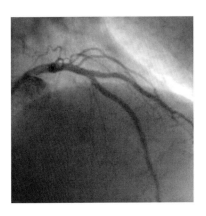
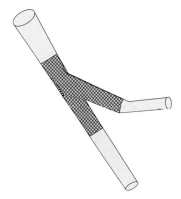

Figure 8 Inverse crushing technique. Final result

REVERSE CRUSHING TECHNIQUE (CASE # 11497/04) (SLIDES 1–11)

(1) Wire branches and pre-dilate
(2) Deploy stent in main branch
(3) Wire side branch and dilate
(4) Position stent in side branch protruding in main branch (slight), leave a balloon in main branch
(5) Deploy stent in side branch and remove wire and balloon
(6) Crush the protruding part of side branch on top of the stent in main branch
(7) Rewire the side branch and perform high-pressure dilatation
(8) Kissing at medium pressure

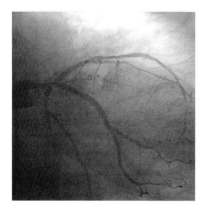
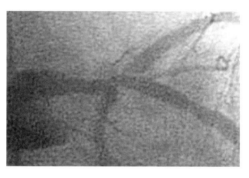

Baseline

Figure 1   Bifurcational stenting 'Reverse crushing'

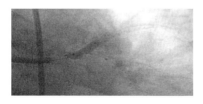
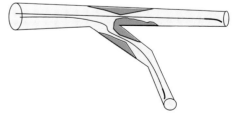

Figure 2   Bifurcational stenting 'Reverse crushing'. Wire both branches and pre-dilate

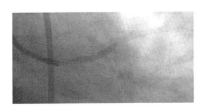
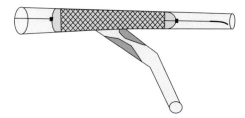

Figure 3   Bifurcational stenting 'Reverse crushing'. Deploy stent in main branch

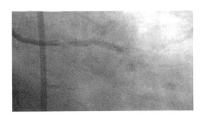
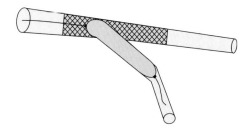

Figure 4   Bifurcational stenting 'Reverse crushing'. Wire side branch and dilate

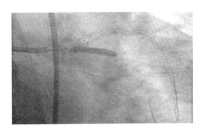
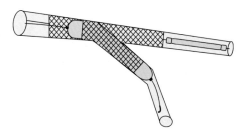

Figure 5   Bifurcational stenting 'Reverse crushing'. Position stent in side branch protruding in MB (slight), leave a balloon in MB and deploy stent in the side branch

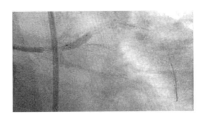
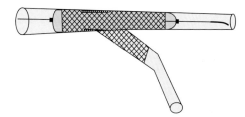

Figure 6   Bifurcational stenting 'Reverse crushing'. Remove wire and balloon from side branch and crush the protruding part of side branch on top of the stent in main branch

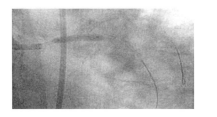
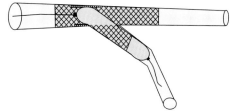

Figure 7 Bifurcational stenting 'Reverse crushing'. Rewire the side branch and perform high-pressure dilatation

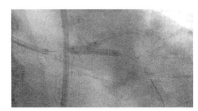
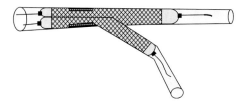

Figure 8 Bifurcational stenting 'Reverse crushing'. Kissing at medium pressure

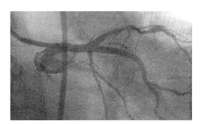
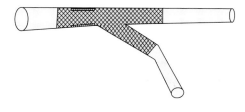

Figure 9 Bifurcational stenting 'Reverse crushing'. Final result

Laboratory insights with different techniques of drug-eluting stent implantation in bifurcations

John Ormiston MD

Slide 2: Introduction

A common method of bifurcation stenting has been to stent the main branch, then using simultaneous ('kissing') balloons to post-dilate the stent, treat the side-branch ostium and correct distortion.

If the side-branch needed stenting, then 'T' stenting has been the most common strategy.

Slide 3: Case # 1

Stenting of the main branch with a drug-eluting stent followed by kissing balloon treatment of the main branch and of the side-branch ostium.

Slide 4

A 61-year-old man presented with angina at rest.

There was a critical left anterior descending stenosis immediately proximal to the major diagonal.

The ostium of the diagonal was only mildly diseased.

The treatment strategy chosen was to stent the LAD across the diagonal then post-dilate with kissing balloons.

If the diagonal result was unsatisfactory after this, the fall-back strategy to treat the diagonal was to be 'internal' (or 'reverse' crushing).

Slide 5

A BMW guide wire (Guidant) was advanced to the diagonal vessel (blue arrow) and another to LAD (red arrow).

LAD was pre-dilated with a 2.5×10-mm balloon (panel A).

A cine (panel B) was recorded with the pre-dilating balloon *in situ* to estimate lesion length (markers are separated by 10-mm).

Slide 6

A. The 3×16-mm Taxus paclitaxel-eluting stent was deployed in LAD (panel A) across the diagonal origin.

B. The resulting diagonal ostial stenosis persisted following intracoronary nitroglycerin (arrow).

C. The diagonal wire had been intentionally 'trapped' between the stent and LAD wall (panel C) when the stent was deployed. This makes wiring of the diagonal through the side of the LAD stent easier.

Slide 7 (**Figure 1**)

A. Shown is the diagonal wire between the stent and LAD vessel wall. This guide wire facilitates guide wire access through the side of the stent to the diagonal.

B. The LAD guide wire was advanced through the side of the stent to the diagonal.

C. The diagonal wire which was between the stent and vessel wall was withdrawn.

D. The diagonal wire was then advanced to LAD.

Slide 8

In panel A, a 1.5-mm diameter balloon is inflated across the side of the stent to separate struts and allow passage of a larger balloon.

In panel B, kissing (simultaneous) post-dilatation was performed using a 3×10-mm balloon in the LAD and a 3.5×10-mm balloon in the diagonal.

Slide 9: **The importance of kissing balloon post-dilatation**

In panel A, the stent was distorted by side-branch balloon dilatation (white arrow). The stent beyond the side branch is narrowed.

In panel B, the distortion was corrected by kissing balloon post-dilatation (black arrow). In addition, the side-branch ostial size is retained.

A Shown is the diagonal wire between the stent and LAD vessel wall. This guide wire facilitates guide wire access through the side of the stent to the diagonal

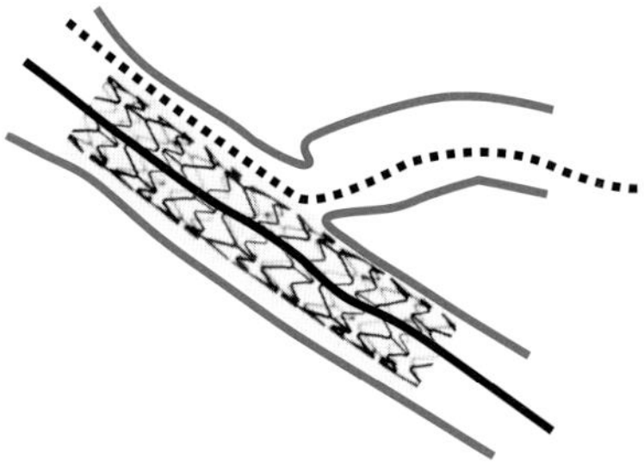

B The LAD guide wire was advanced through the side of the stent to the diagonal

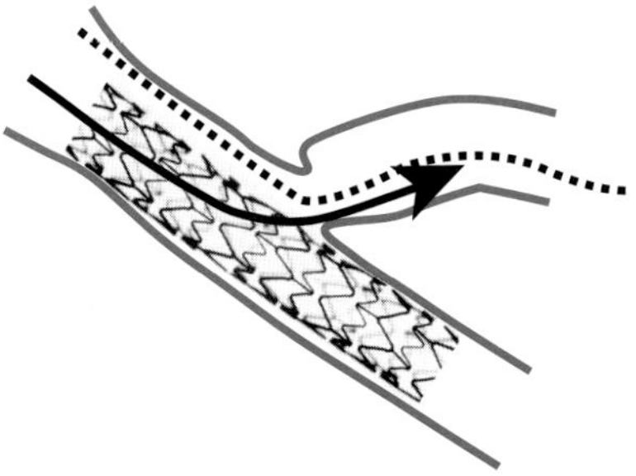

C The diagonal wire which was between the stent and vessel wall was withdrawn

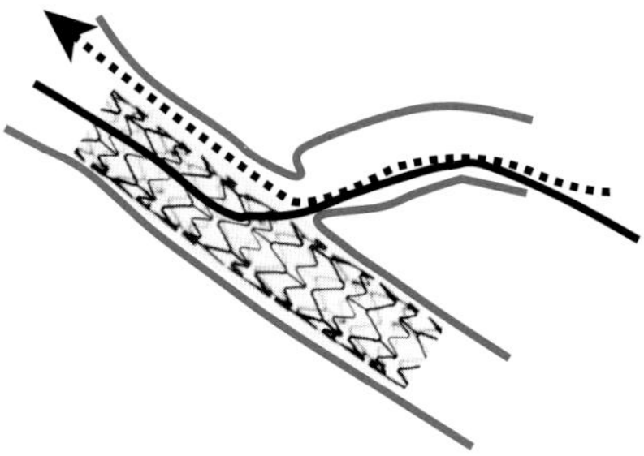

D The 'diagonal' wire was then advanced to LAD

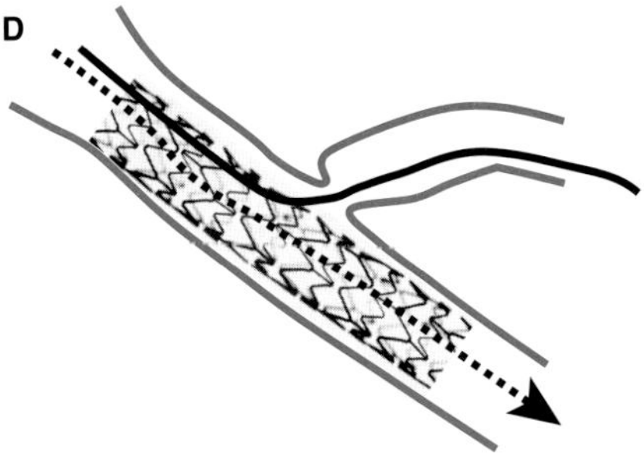

Figure 1

Slide 10

The final result after Taxus stent deployment (broken line indicates the length of the stent) and kissing balloon post-dilatation is excellent with full caliber at the diagonal ostium (arrow). There was no need for side-branch stenting.

Slide 11: **Advantages and limitation of single stent deployment for bifurcations**

Stenting the main branch with balloon treatment of the side branch produced an excellent result in Case 1.

Outcomes when only one drug-eluting stent is needed are very good.[1]

However in a recent trial of bifurcation stenting with DES, half of those randomized to a single-stent strategy crossed over to receive two DES using the strategy of 'T' stenting.[1]

Slide 12: **Limitations of 'T'-stenting (Figure 2)**

It is very difficult to place the side-branch stent so that there is scaffolding of the side-branch ostium without gaps.

In panel A the stent is too distal so that there are gaps in scaffolding and drug application.

In panel C, the stent is too proximal and potentially obstructs the main.

It may be impossible to pass a stent to the side branch.

Slide 13

Restenoses that occurred when two drug-eluting stents (DES) were used were at the ostium of the side branch (1) and thought to be due to gaps in stent scaffolding and drug application.

This prompted the introduction of the innovative *'crush' technique* (Colombo) that ensures full coverage of the side-branch ostium without gaps in scaffolding or drug delivery especially if kissing balloon post-dilatation is performed.[1]

Slide 14

The basic external crush technique is:

• Simple
• Safe (wire access to branches is retained until stents deployed)
• Limits ischemic time (important in e.g. left main stenting)

Limitations of 'T'-stenting

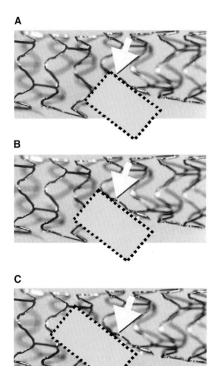

A

B

C

- It is very difficult to place the side-branch stent so that there is scaffolding of the side-branch ostium without gaps

- In panel A the stent is too distal so that there are gaps in scaffolding and drug application

- In panel C, the stent is too proximal and potentially obstructs the main

- It may be impossible to pass a stent to the side branch

Figure 2

Slide 15

Kissing balloon post-dilatation:

- Fully expands the stent at the side-branch ostium
- Partially releases the side branch from jail facilitating subsequent side-branch access
- Is the most difficult part of the procedure

Slide 16

The next slides describe how to carry out bifurcation stenting using the 'external crush' technique plus post-dilatation with simultaneous kissing balloon inflations.

Slide 17

Pass wires to both branches.

Predilate one branch. Ensure that balloon length is shorter than intended DES length.

Predilate the other branch.

Slide 18

Position the DES (yellow) to be crushed partially in the side branch and partially in the main branch. Ensure that the main branch stent (blue) extends more proximally than the side-branch stent.

Deploy the side-branch stent and remove the deploying balloon. Administer intracoronary nitroglycerin and repeat angiography before the side-branch wire is removed. This may be the last chance to treat dissection distal to the side-branch stent.

Remove the wire from the side branch before deploying the main branch stent.

Slide 19

Deploy the main branch stent crushing that portion of the side-branch stent within the main branch.

Cross with a wire (PT Graphics or Sport) through the two layers of stent that separate the main branch lumen from the side-branch lumen. Predilate the side-branch with e.g. a 1.5-mm Maverick balloon (Boston Scientific).

Post-dilate using simultaneous kissing balloons.

Slide 20

The final result after crushing and kissing. The side-branch ostium is fully expanded without gaps in scaffolding or drug application.

The three layers of stent (*) just proximal to the side branch are visible on angiography as an increased radiodensity and have been mistaken for intimal dissection.

Slide 21: **Tips to help with kissing balloon post-dilatation (the most challenging part of the procedure) (Figure 3)**

Use a very stiff wire (e.g. Sport, Guidant). If this fails to cross, try a PT Graphics wire (Boston Scientific).

**Tips to help with kissing balloon post-dilatation
(the most challenging part of the procedure)**

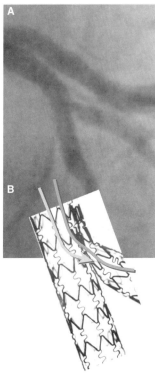

- Use a very stiff wire (e.g. Sport, Guidant). If this fails to cross, try a PT Graphics wire (Boston Scientific)

- Use a 1.5-mm Maverick balloon (Boston Scientific) to separate struts and allow a larger balloon to pass to the side branch

If balloon won't cross:

- Rewire the side branch. A different course may be followed through the two layers of stent separating the main and side branches

- Post-dilate the main branch stent. This may separate struts enough to pass a 1.5-mm balloon

Balloon inflations:

- Inflate both balloons simultaneously and slowly. This makes 'melon seeding' less likely

- Deflate the balloons simultaneously to avoid distortion

Figure 3

Use a 1.5-mm Maverick balloon (Boston Scientific) to separate struts and allow a larger balloon to pass to the side branch.

If balloon won't cross:

- Rewire the side branch. A different course may be followed through the two layers of stent separating the main and side branches
- Post-dilate the main branch stent. This may separate struts enough to pass a 1.5-mm balloon

Balloon inflations:

- Inflate both balloons simultaneously and slowly. This makes 'melon seeding' less likely
- Deflate the balloons simultaneously to avoid distortion

Slide 22

We have bench tested the crush technique with the Bx Velocity and Express[2] stents that are the delivery platforms for the Cypher sirolimus-eluting and Taxus paclitaxel-eluting systems, respectively.

Bench performance with other designs may be different.

Slide 23: **Case # 2**

A bifurcation stenosis treated with two Taxus stents using the crush technique followed by kissing balloon post-dilatation.

Slide 24

Mrs K, an 80-year-old woman was admitted with Braunwald class III unstable angina.

Coronary angiography revealed a severe bifurcation stenosis involving the left anterior descending (LAD) and major diagonal (diag) arteries (type 1 bifurcation lesion).

The ostium of the diagonal had important stenosis. There was a high chance that the side branch would become occluded or more severely narrowed if LAD alone were stented.

Slide 25: **Crush technique continued**

Through an 8-Fr JL3.5 guide catheter, a BMW guide wire (Guidant) was passed to each branch.

A 2.5×10-mm CrossSail balloon was used to predilate the LAD (*frame A*), then diagonal (*frame B*).

Pre-dilating balloon length is shorter than planned drug-eluting stent length.

Panel C is the angiogram after pre-dilatation and intracoronary nitroglycerin.

Slide 26

A 3×12-mm Taxus stent was passed to the diagonal vessel (red arrows) and a 3×20-mm Taxus stent was passed to the LAD (blue arrows).

The length of artery exposed to pre-dilatation will be covered by stent.

The portion of diagonal stent in the LAD will be crushed and completely covered by the LAD stent.

In panel B, the diagonal Taxus stent is deployed at 14 atm.

Slide 27

The guide wire and balloon were removed from the diagonal vessel (panel A). Note that the ostium of the diagonal has no stenosis (black arrow).

Then the 3×20-mm Taxus stent was deployed in the LAD at 14 atm (panel B). This crushed that portion of the diagonal stent in the LAD.

Slide 28

Following deployment of the LAD Taxus stent, stenosis appeared at the diagonal ostium.

This was probably due to distortion of the crushed stent (red arrows in bench photograph). In addition plaque shift may play a role.

Circled is the crushed stent (three layers).

There are two layers of stent between the LAD and diagonal.

Slide 29

A PT Graphics wire was passed through two layers of stent into the side-branch as shown on the bench (A).

Then a 1.5-mm Maverick balloon (Boston Scientific) was inflated across the struts.

After this, a 3×10-mm Crossail balloon was inflated in the diagonal simultaneously (B) with an identical balloon in the LAD to 14 atm (kissing balloon post-dilatation).

Care was taken to deflate the balloons simultaneously.

Kissing balloons fully expand the side-branch stent at the ostium and partially release the side-branch from jail (C).

Slide 30

The final result after deployment of two Taxus stents in the bifurcation using the crush technique and kissing balloon post-dilatation. A very good result is achieved with good expansion of the side-branch ostium.

Slide 31

Kissing balloon post-dilatation can cause stent distortion if improperly performed.

Stent distortion from improperly performed kissing balloon post-dilatation

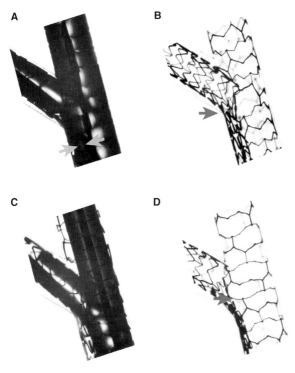

- In panel A, the main vessel kissing balloon is smaller than the deploying balloon. This caused distortion of the stents (blue arrow, panel B)

- In panel C, the main vessel kissing balloon was the same size or larger than the deploying balloon and there was no distortion (panel D)

Figure 4

Slide 32: Stent distortion from improperly performed kissing balloon post-dilatation (Figure 4)

In panel A, the main vessel kissing balloon is smaller than the deploying balloon. This caused distortion of the stents (blue arrow, panel B).

In panel C, the main vessel kissing balloon was the same size or larger than the deploying balloon and there was no distortion (panel D).

Slide 33: Case # 3

'Internal' or 'reverse' crush provisional side-branch stenting strategy.

Slide 34

The crush technique has many advantages but is a commitment to stenting both branches and to using two drug-eluting stents.

If a single drug-eluting stent can be deployed in the main branch without the need for side-branch stenting, adequate immediate and long-term outcomes can be achieved.[1]

However if a single drug-eluting stent is deployed in the main branch, there needs to be a safe reliable strategy to stent the side branch if necessary.

In addition, the side-branch stent needs to be fully expanded so that there is full scaffolding and drug application to the side-branch ostium where most restenoses occur.

Slide 35

The 'internal' or 'reverse' crush technique is such a provisonal side-branch stenting strategy.

It allows stenting of the side branch with full ostial scaffolding and drug application.

Its major limitation is that it may not be impossible to pass a stent across the side of the main branch stent so there is a potential for failure to adequately treat the side-branch.

Slide 36

The drug-eluting stenting strategy planned for this patient was to deliver a long stent to the LAD, then carry out kissing balloon post-dilatation.

If the side branch needed stenting, then 'internal' (or 'reverse') crushing was planned.

'T' stenting was not entertained as a strategy because of the problem of gaps and difficulty fully scaffolding the side-branch ostium.

Slide 37 (**Figure 5**)

A 3×33-mm sirolimus-eluting stent was deployed in the LAD.

A stenosis unresponsive to intracoronary nitroglycerin appeared at the ostium of the diagonal (arrows).

Slide 38

The diagonal ostial stenosis persisted (panel B) after kissing balloon inflations (panel A).

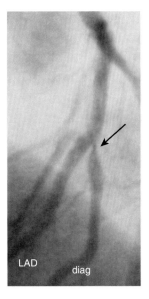 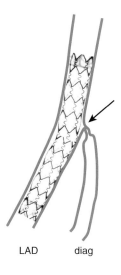

- A 3 × 33-mm sirolimus-eluting stent was deployed in the LAD

- A stenosis unresponsive to intracoronary nitroglycerin appeared at the ostium of the diagonal (arrows)

Figure 5

Slide 39 (Figure 6)

An undeployed balloon is 'parked' inside the LAD sirolimus-eluting stent.

A second sirolimus-eluting stent (S) is passed part-way the side of the LAD stent into the side branch.

Slide 40 (Figure 7)

The side-branch stent (sb) is deployed so that it lies partly within the LAD stent and partly in the diagonal branch.

The undeployed balloon (b) lies within the LAD stent.

Slide 41 (Figure 8)

The balloon that had been 'parked' in the LAD stent is expanded so that it crushes the side-branch stent inside the LAD stent (arrow).

This contrasts with the conventional external crush technique where the stent is crushed outside the LAD stent.

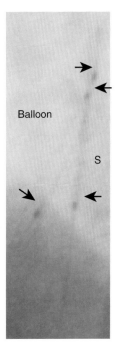 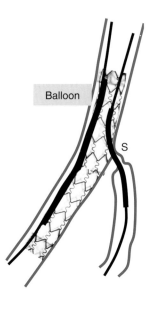

- An undeployed balloon is 'parked' inside the LAD sirolimus-eluting stent

- A second sirolimus-eluting stent (S) is passed part-way the side of the LAD stent into the side branch

Figure 6

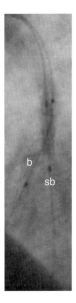 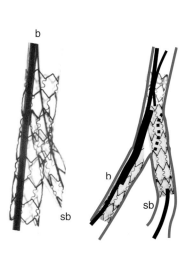

- The side-branch stent (sb) is deployed so that it lies partly within the LAD stent and partly in the diagonal branch

- The undeployed balloon (b) lies within the LAD stent

Figure 7

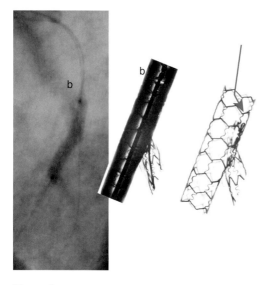

- The balloon that had been 'parked' in the LAD stent is expanded so that it crushes the side-branch stent inside the LAD stent (arrow)

- This contrasts with the conventional external crush technique where the stent is crushed outside the LAD stent

Figure 8

Slide 42

In the left panel is the angiographic outcome at the completion of the internal crush procedure.

In the right panel is the result at 1 year after implantation showing an excellent late result.

Slide 43: Summary

The 'external crush' technique for bifurcation stenting with DES ensures coverage of the side-branch ostium without gaps.

Kissing balloon post-dilatation after 'external crush' ensures best scaffolding and drug application, releases the side branch from jail, and can correct distortion.

If a single DES is deployed, there needs to be a safe reliable way to stent the side branch with full ostial scaffolding and drug application.

Slide 44

Provisional side-branch stenting strategies that cover the ostium without gaps include the 'internal crush' technique.

Undersized main branch kissing balloon after 'external crush' (and 'culotte') stenting causes stent distortion.

After 'internal crush' paradoxically any kissing balloon post-dilatation causes distortion.

REFERENCE

1. Colombo A, Moses JW, Morice ME, et al. Randomized study to evaluate sirolimuseluting stents implanted at coronary bifurcation lesions. Circulation 2004; 109: 1244–9

Complex Lesions
Part II – Very Long Lesions

1. Enhanced drug delivery with sonotherapy treatment

Case # 11005/02

Case # 11005/02 is illustrated by **slides 1–9** (*frames 1–21*). This is a diabetic patient with a long diffused disease of the left anterior descending involving a bifurcation with a diagonal branch. The patient was treated with multiple Cypher-stent (Cordis) implantation to cover extensively the left anterior descending and the crush technique was performed at the level of the diagonal branch. *Frame 7* shows a residual dissection, which was treated by additional Cypher-stent implantation. At the end of the procedure, the entire proximal and mid-LAD is covered by Cypher stents as demonstrated in *frame 9*. At that time, part of the sonotherapy research protocol was performed to improve the drug delivery in a subset of patients with diabetes in which the results with drug-eluting stents were still sub-optimal. The final result, following sonotherapy delivered only on the LAD, is shown in *frames 12* and *13*. The procedure was continued on the same patient by treating three lesions in the right coronary artery with implantation of three Cypher stents. Again, this vessel was treated with sonotherapy. The follow-up result shows excellent patency of the left anterior descending. There was a very focal stenosis at the ostium of the diagonal branch, while the right coronary artery is also widely patent.

Message The disappearance of sonotherapy did not allow testing the concept of enhanced drug delivery in high-risk patients.

2. A severely calcified lesion: importance of rotational atherectomy

Case # 11608/03

Case # 11608/03 is illustrated by **slides 1–5** (*frames 1–12*). This is a patient with diffuse disease and calcific lesions in the right coronary artery. The images of multiple filling defects are suggestive of calcification. The only differential diagnosis in this circumstance is with multiple thrombotic lesions, which are distinguished mainly by the clinical presentation. *Frames 1* and *2* illustrate the baseline situation in the right coronary artery.

Owing to the extensive calcification, the vessel was pretreated with rotational atherectomy (1.5-mm burr). Notice the presence of a pacemaker wire in the right ventricle. Following rotablation, the vessel was dilated with a 2.5-mm balloon; it is always important to perform low-pressure balloon dilatation following rotablation to improve the distal flow and to remove some spasm. Three Taxus stents (Boston Scientific) were then deployed in the right coronary artery as shown in *frames 8, 9* and *10*. The final result is presented in *frames 11* and *12*, with excellent expansion of the stent.

Message   We believe that in diffuse disease, particularly with calcified lesions, the rule of appropriate and full vessel preparation should be very carefully followed in order to achieve stent delivery, optimal stent expansion, and drug delivery to the vessel wall.

3. IVUS evaluation for long diffuse disease treatment

Case # 11761/03

Case # 11761/03 is illustrated by **slides 1–6** (*frames 1–15*). This is a patient with diffuse disease of a small obtuse marginal branch highlighted by multiple arrows in *frames 1* and *2*. The vessel was first pre-dilated with an Fx Minirail 2.5 mm (Guidant). Following pre-dilatation, the vessel appears significantly larger. In order to better evaluate the true diameter of this vessel, intravascular ultrasound was performed as demonstrated in *frames 5, 6* and *7*. The vessel diameter at the level of the distal obtuse marginal branch is, according to IVUS, 2.5 mm – measuring the diameter from media to media. For this reason, a 2.5-mm Cypher stent was selected. In the more intermediate part of the vessel, the IVUS measurements corresponded to 3 mm in diameter, and a 3-mm Cypher stent was selected. Moving more proximally, the haziness present on angiography corresponded to a large plaque with a stenosis of 73%, as shown in *frame 8*. For this reason, a large 3.5-mm Cypher stent was selected to be implanted at this level. The final result is demonstrated in *frames 10* and *11*, with IVUS control in *frames 12–15*. It is rewarding to see the optimal result achieved in this vessel, thanks to appropriate selection of three different stents, appropriately sized.

Message   In the context of diffuse disease, IVUS evaluation is the best tool for selecting the most appropriately sized stent. It will allow negative remodeling to be distinguished from large plaque burden, and ultimately the right stent to be implanted without the risk of undersizing in order to avoid vessel rupture (or, alternatively, to do the opposite, with the risk of vessel rupture). In the context of diffuse disease, it is not rare to see segments with no or negative remodeling and areas with marked positive remodeling.

4. Atherectomy and DES: is it needed?

Case # 11812/03

This is a case (**slides 1–7** (*frames 1–16*)) of diffuse disease of the circumflex. The lesion involves the bifurcation of the obtuse marginal branch and the postero-lateral branch. *Frames 1* and *2* demonstrate the baseline lesion. Following lesion pre-dilatation as shown in *frames 3–5*, the procedure was completed with atherectomy utilizing a Silverhawk catheter from Foxhollow. The results after atherectomy are presented in *frame 7*. Following this procedure, Taxus stents were implanted according to the crush technique to cover the ostium of the obtuse marginal and postero-lateral branch. Stents were also implanted in the proximal part of the circumflex. Final kissing balloon inflation was performed as shown in *frame 11*, with the result of the crush technique demonstrated in *frame 12*. A more proximal Taxus stent was then implanted following pre-dilatation of the other obtuse marginal branch with the cutting balloon. The final result is presented in *frames 15* and *16*.

Message   The remarkable final minimal lumen diameter (MLD) achieved when a combination of atherectomy and stent implantation is performed is clear. The optimal synergy is when a drug-eluting stent is utilized. The unsolved question is to what level of complexity of lesion preparation we need to go to optimize the immediate and the follow-up results of drug-eluting stent implantation.

COMPLEX LESIONS
PART III – SMALL VESSELS

1. Multiple stents in a small vessel

Case # 9691/2000

This case (slides 1–7 (*frames 1–20*)) illustrates a focal lesion in the obtuse marginal branch of the circumflex followed by an area of diffuse disease. The original plan was to cover this lesion with a single 2.5×18-mm stent. This task was effectively achieved as demonstrated in *frame 5*. Owing to the presence of diffuse disease and concerns regarding the outflow tract of this stent, a second stent of the same length and diameter was implanted. The presence of a hinge effect at the level of the distal second stent then prompted implantation of a third 18-mm stent. The final result is demonstrated in *frame 11*. The interesting part of this case is that at the 6-month follow-up, there was almost no late loss, as demonstrated in *frame 14*. The IVUS evaluation confirms the angiographic appearance. *Frames 15, 16* and *17* not only demonstrate the presence of minimal or no hyperplasia, but they show this fact despite the presence of a grossly under-expanded stent in *frames 16* and *17*. This result at 6 months was fully maintained at 36 months despite discontinuation of double anti-platelet therapy, which was implemented after 6-month treatment owing to multiple stent implantations.

Message   This case represents another example of the almost complete abolition of late loss, even in small vessels with the stent underdeployed.

2. Three bifurcations, a total occlusion, and small vessels with long diseased segment

Case # 10856/02

This is a case (slides 1–10 (*frames 1–25*)) that illustrates several issues, including: total occlusions, small vessels, and several bifurcations.
    Frame 1 illustrates the baseline angiogram in the RAO-cranial projection and *frame 2* in the LAO-cranial. From this view, the left anterior descending (LAD) is

occluded following the origin of two diagonal branches. We can assume that the LAD is not going to be a large vessel, due to the fact that the vessel is basically composed of three branches: the LAD and two diagonal branches. The longer arrows point to the occlusion of the LAD, and the shorter arrows to the several diseased areas in a diagonal branch. The LAD occlusion was successfully crossed with a wire as illustrated in *frame 4*. Another diagonal branch was then wired in the more distal part of the LAD. This diagonal was pre-dilated as shown in *frame 5* and then immediately secured with implantation of two stents: one in the LAD and the other in the diagonal according to the crush technique (*frames 6* and *7*). First inflation of the diagonal-branch stent was carried out, and then of the LAD stent, after removal of wire and balloon from the diagonal. *Frame 8* shows the result in the distal LAD with maintained patency of the diagonal branch. In complex lesions such as this, this approach may significantly simplify the procedure.

The operator then concentrated on the second bifurcation, which is the LAD and the second diagonal branch. The lesion was treated according to the crush technique as shown in *frame 9*. In this *frame*, the two stents appeared satisfactorily deployed with an adequate protrusion of the stent in the diagonal to the LAD. In reality, the severe angulation of the diagonal misled the operator and, as will be noticed later, the ostium of the diagonal was not fully covered. *Frames 10* and *11* illustrate the performance of the crush technique, and *frame 12* presents the final result in the cranial projection, which shows an apparent good coverage of the diagonal origin. The operator then decided to treat the more distal LAD, which appeared still narrowed: a small Cypher 2.25 × 18-mm stent (Cordis) was implanted. The result in the distal LAD is presented in *frame 15*. Notice excellent patency of the diagonal branch. In *frame 16*, it is now apparent that the ostium of the second diagonal was not fully covered; there is a clear gap between the LAD and the diagonal stent. For this reason, POBA was performed, and a short Cypher stent was inserted in the diagonal to cover the gap (*frame 18*). *Frame 19* shows residual disease, which was not yet treated in the first diagonal branch. This vessel was pre-dilated as shown in *frame 20*, and then a Cypher 2.25 × 33-mm stent was inserted in this branch. The stent is positioned in order to be relatively precise to the ostium as shown in *frame 21* (T-stenting), while leaving a wire in the LAD. The LAD was not stented because, at this level, the vessel appeared without significant disease. *Frames 22* and *23* demonstrate the final result. More rewarding is the 8-month angiographic follow-up which showed sustained patency with no restenosis in any of the branches treated. It is worth mentioning that final kissing in the crush bifurcation was performed only in the lesion in the intermediate diagonal and not in the distal diagonal.

Message   The main message of this case is the superb performance of these stents even in complex lesions in small vessels and in multiple bifurcations. The long stents appear to defeat the prior assumption that the restenosis rate is dependent on the stent length.

3. A long segment with diffuse disease

Case # 11195/02

This is an example (**slides 1–4** (*frames 1–9*)) of a long lesion in a very small vessel involving a long segment of an acute marginal branch distributing as posterior descending or postero-lateral branch of the right coronary artery. *Frame 1* illustrates the baseline segment of diffused disease. As always in these long segments, pre-dilatation is very important in order to better evaluate the true size of the vessel and decide the appropriate stent size to be used. As a matter of fact, following pre-dilatation, the distal vessel appears large enough to accept a 2.5-mm stent. This stent is implanted as shown in *frame 5*. A 33-mm-long stent is used. Owing to the presence of significant diffuse disease, an additional stent was added, 2.25 × 18 mm long, as demonstrated in *frame 7*. The final result is shown in *frame 8* and the follow-up, almost identical, is shown in *frame 9*.

Message   This is another example of excellent performance of long stents in small vessels without significant late loss, despite the association of the two most common variables creating late loss: small reference-vessel size and long stent implantation.

4. Small vessel with severe calcification, tortuosity, and subtotal occlusion

Case # 11895/04

This case (**slides 1–4** (*frames 1–7* and *runs 1, 2*)) illustrates a lesion with severe calcification, tortuosity and subtotal occlusion involving the obtuse marginal branch. *Run 1* and still *frame 1* demonstrate this lesion with faint visualization of the distal obtuse marginal branch. The lesion was crossed utilizing a hydrophilic wire and then careful lesion preparation was performed combining cutting balloon and POBA. The result before stenting is illustrated in *frame 4*. It is very important in this tortuous vessel to be sure that the lesion is appropriately prepared before advancing the stent in order to facilitate stent advancement and optimal stent implantation. A 2.5 × 33-mm Cypher stent is advanced in this tortuous anatomy with appropriate positioning (*frame 5*). The final result is demonstrated in *run 2*.

Summaries of the case are shown in *frame 6*, with the final result presented in *frame 7*.

Message   The main message of this case is the value of lesion preparation in order to allow the advancement of a long stent in a tortuous vessel.

5. Skipping a bifurcation in a small vessel with diffuse disease

Case # 11911/04

This is an example (**slides 1–3** (*frames 1–7*)) of a long lesion involving a very distal bifurcation on a small intermediate branch. *Frame 1* illustrates the baseline
lesion, which originates from a distal bifurcation of an intermediate branch. The
lesion is pre-dilated and then a 2.25 × 28-mm Cypher stent is deployed right proximal to the bifurcation. In these small bifurcations, an attempt is frequently made not
to stent the bifurcation. The final result is demonstrated in *frame 7*.

Message   The main message of this case is that, in relatively small vessels, a
strategy which is aimed to simplify the procedure is necessary: trying to stent the
main part of the small vessel and leaving the side branches open – possibly without
additional stenting.

COMPLEX LESIONS
PART IV – OSTIAL LESIONS

1. Ostial circumflex or unprotected left main stenting

Case # 11585/03

This is a typical situation, which brings with it controversies regarding the best way to approach this type of lesion (**slides 1–6** (*frames 1–13*)). A lesion involving the ostial part of the circumflex, and in this case being more complex, involving a bifurcation of the circumflex, represents a challenge with regards to the most appropriate approach.

Unfortunately, this controversy is not easy to settle because we lack any scientific data, and most of the suggestions come from personal experience and anecdotal cases.

There are, in general, two lines of approach. First, the extensive stenting approach in which both branches, including the left main, are stented with the idea to reconstruct the trifurcation. Second, a more conservative approach in which only the most diseased vessel is stented, trying to limit stenting to the ostium and performing provisional angioplasty on the other branches. In this specific case, we decided to perform extensive stenting.

As I said at the beginning, the fact that we decided to adopt this technique does not necessarily imply that this technique is the best. What is important to keep in mind is that if the interventionist decides to perform extensive stenting, the only stents that can be used are drug-eluting stents.

Frames 1 and *2* show the baseline lesion, which is mainly confined to the ostial and proximal part of the true circumflex; there is some modest disease in the distal segment of the left main.

Following wiring of the two branches (circumflex and LAD) and pre-dilatation, two stents are positioned with the crush approach, stenting the left main towards the LAD and the true circumflex, which becomes the crushed vessel. Stent positioning is shown in *frame 3*, and *frame 4* shows the results, which show a compromise of the ostial portion of the intermediate branch.

Frame 5 shows pre-dilatation of the ostium of the intermediate branch and then placement of a Cypher stent at this level, with the idea to crush this stent towards the LAD. Other protective balloons are positioned in the LAD and in the true circumflex, in order to crush the protruding part of the stent in the ramus. Following deployment of the stenting ramus, *frame 8* shows partial compromise of the ostial portion of the left anterior descending. The branches are then wired and balloons are inflated, first separately then simultaneously (*frame 9*). The final result is demonstrated in *frames 10* and *11*. It is obvious that the branches are all widely patent, in particular the left main. Follow-up angiogram demonstrated persistent optimal stent patency (*frames 12* and *13*).

Message   Unfortunately, we do not know whether this complex approach is the best solution. It is clearly the approach that gives the best immediate results and, if we have the luxury of using a stent with no restenosis, it should be the approach which maintains the best long-term result.

2. Use of debulking in a very proximal lesion

Case # 11609/03

This is a typical case (**slides 1–4** (*frames 1–8*)), which illustrates classic treatment of an ostial left anterior descending lesion in a patient who failed coronary artery by-pass grafting. This very proximal left anterior descending lesion with some diffuse disease in the mid-portion of the vessel is first treated with debulking in order to minimize plaque shift towards the circumflex. This technique, in our view, still has value in very proximal and ostial left anterior descending lesions and in selected circumflex lesions.

Following directional atherectomy, which can also be performed with the Flexicut (Guidant) atherectomy catheter, the result is demonstrated in *frame 4*. A Taxus stent, 3.5×16 mm long, is then implanted proximally, and then another stent is implanted in the mid-part. It is clear that the final results, as shown in *frames 7* and *8*, do not show any compromise of the circumflex. These results, were obtained without the need to perform kissing inflation towards the circumflex.

Message   The main message of this case is the value of the selective use of debulking techniques in very proximal lesions, particularly when plaque shift needs to be minimized.

3. Crush stenting for ostial LAD lesion

Case # 11645/03

This is an example of an ostial LAD lesion (**slides 1–5** (*frames 1–10* and *runs 1–3*)), which again could be treated in a number of ways. It depends on the experience of the operator with this particular type of lesion. *Run 1* shows an IVUS baseline evaluation at the level of the left anterior descending, which demonstrates some moderate calcifications. The approach here could be to perform first atherectomy, perhaps with the Foxhollow system. The operator decided to proceed with a crush technique, with positioning of a stent in the circumflex in order to protect plaque shift and compression of this vessel.

In our experience, when the origin is more V-type like the one demonstrated in *frame 2*, the risk of compressing the circumflex following stenting of the LAD is significant. Another possibility would be to implant two stents according to the V-technique. *Frame 3* shows the implantation of the two stents with inflation first of the stent in the circumflex (*Frame 4*), then inflation of the stent in the left anterior descending. Rewiring of the circumflex is demonstrated in *frame 6*, and the final kissing balloon is demonstrated in *frame 7*.

The final result is shown in *frame 9*. There is wide patency of the left anterior descending, with minimal residual narrowing at the ostium of the circumflex. Despite this angiographically imperfect result (as shown in *frame 10*), the IVUS run in the circumflex did not show any compromise at the ostium of this vessel, and no further actions were taken. In the same slide, we see the IVUS run in the LAD, which demonstrates an optimal final result.

Message   It is difficult to make a final statement regarding the best technique to employ in these ostial lesions. As said at the beginning, atherectomy with provisional stenting in the circumflex and stenting of the LAD, is certainly another choice. V-stenting of the bifurcation is again a second choice, and the one we demonstrated here is a third choice.

4. A trifurcation of the left main with severe calcifications: provisional stenting on the intermediate branch

Case # 11244/03

This case (**slides 1–6** (*frames 1–18*)) illustrates treatment of two ostial lesions that are severely calcified, involving the ostium of the circumflex and of the intermediate branch. Baseline lesions are shown in *frames 1* and *2*. It is important to notice that sometimes these lesions may demand treatment of the left main in order to obtain a good final result. Owing to severe calcification of the vessels, pre-dilatation was performed (with a standard balloon to allow cutting balloon passage), then with a cutting balloon, and completed with a high-pressure balloon inflated up to 30 atm. These steps are shown in *frames 3–6*. The final result following pre-dilatation in the intermediate branch is shown in *frame 7*. The operator then addressed the circumflex. Pre-dilatation showed that it was impossible to fully expand the balloon. An attempt to cross the lesion with a cutting balloon (as shown in *frame 9*) failed, and the operator utilized rotational atherectomy as shown in *frame 10*. Following rotablation, a cutting balloon inflation was performed, and the more distal part of the vessel was treated with a 2.5-mm balloon as shown in *frame 11*. *Frame 12* shows the result in the circumflex. The decision was then taken to stent the circumflex and the LAD while trying to maintain patency with balloon inflation of the intermediate branch. Two Cypher stents were positioned according to the crush technique as shown in *frames 13* and *14*.

The result after stenting the circumflex is shown in *frame 15*, and then deployment of the stent in the LAD is shown in *frame 16*. The final result is shown in *frame 17*, with stenting of the left main and preservation of the intermediate branch, which in this case was not stented (*frames 17* and *18*).

Message   It is always very important to prepare the lesion well, particularly when the lesion is severely calcified.

5. A typical ostial LAD lesion

Case # 11795/03

This is a typical example (**slides 1–6** (*frames 1–12*)) of an ostial lesion of the left anterior descending, which brings into attention several problems – among them appropriate stent positioning. *Frames 1* and *2* show the baseline lesion in the proximal and ostial LAD. The stent is positioned in *frame 3* with the marker, which appears to be in the left main. The deployment is shown in *frame 4*. Following deployment, *frames 5* and *6* clearly illustrate that the ostium was not fully covered. This situation is most probably explained by the profound foreshortening that the LAD has in the caudal LAO projection. It is always important to check the positioning of the stent in two orthogonal projections. The other projections we suggest are a caudal RAO or, in some situations, a cranial RAO. The next step at this point was to place a stent covering partially the left main as shown in *frame 7*. The final result in *frame 9* shows some plaque shift towards the circumflex, which was corrected by kissing inflation as shown in *frame 10*. The very final result is demonstrated in *frames 11* and *12*.

Message   Despite an attempt not to cover the left main when stenting the ostial LAD, sometimes this problem cannot be completely avoided and stenting into the left main becomes necessary. If a partial compromise of the circumflex occurs, it is always important to try first with a simple balloon dilatation before going into another stent implantation into the circumflex, which should only be reserved for a clear suboptimal result.

COMPLEX LESIONS
PART V – CHRONIC TOTAL OCCLUSIONS

1. Complex in-stent chronic total occlusion

Case # 10750/02

Case # 10750/02 is illustrated by **slides 1–5** (*frames 1–7* and *runs 1–3*). This case represents an occlusion, intra-stent, of a dominant right coronary artery as demonstrated in *frames 1* and *2*. The patient underwent several attempts to reopen the diffuse intra-stent occlusion without success. During the last attempt, utilization of the Frontrunner (LuMend) allowed its negotiation up to the distal part of the lesion. *Frames 4* and *5* show the Frontrunner, which now has reached the most distal stent. We believe that this device is particularly suitable for stent occlusion because the large profile of the device allows it to stay inside the stent channel. The result following the first passage of the Frontrunner is presented in *frame 2*. There is still occlusion at the distal part of the most distal stent, which was successfully negotiated with a wire. Following extensive pre-dilatation, six Cypher stents were implanted to fully cover the diseased right coronary artery. The final result is presented in *run 3* and *frame 7*. The patient was asymptomatic at 1-year follow-up.

Message The Frontrunner appears to be a useful device to cross complex in-stent total occlusions with a better guarantee of maintaining an intra-stent position. Under these conditions, a full metal jacket with drug-eluting stents appears appropriate, and usually the long-term results are remarkable.

2. A case of chronic total occlusion with stenting from proximal to distal

Case # 10923/02

This is a case (**slides 1–4** (*frames 1–8*)) of total occlusion of the LAD with an unfavorable anatomy. In *frame 2*, there is a suggestion for a stump. In addition, there is a side branch, which originates at the site of occlusion. The contralateral injection performed from the right coronary artery (demonstrated in *frame 3*) shows that the occlusion is reasonably long from the segment visualized through the collaterals (see arrows). With the help of the contralateral injection and a dedicated wire such as the Conquest (Asahi Intec, Japan), the occlusion was finally crossed, as demonstrated in *frame 4*. Pre-dilatation was performed and then Cypher stent implantation was undertaken. Notice that in this case the first stent was implanted in the proximal part and then more distally. Despite being unconventional, this approach is sometimes utilized in some total occlusions with diffused disease, in order not to overstent the vessel and to better visualize the distal part in order to make an evaluation as to where to place the additional stent. This particular lesion was treated with two stents: one 33 mm in length (*frame 5*) and the other 18 mm in length (*frame 6*). The final results are demonstrated in *frames 7* and *8*.

Message   In some conditions stenting from proximal to distal can be utilized. In our view, this approach should be used very selectively, and we do not recommend it in every or even in most total occlusions. Sometimes it may be very difficult and time consuming to advance a stent distally to a stent that has just been deployed. Despite this limitation, it is important to bear in mind that the approach of stenting from proximal to distal is an option that could be occasionally utilized.

3. Contra-lateral injection and stent implantation from proximal to distal site

Case # 11291/03

This case (**slides 1–4** (*frames 1–11*)) involves an old total occlusion of the left anterior descending after the origin of a diagonal branch.

   The case illustrates the value of contra-lateral injection, taking the benefits of collaterals originating from the right coronary artery (*frame 2*). The lesion was successfully crossed utilizing a Conquest Pro guide-wire (Asahi Intec, Japan) and then balloon dilatation was performed. The contra-lateral injection is of importance to guide advancement of a stiff and pointed wire in the occlusion and to facilitate negotiating this wire in a diffused disease vessel. The result following the first stent implantation is shown in *frame 6*. This stent is a 33-mm-long Cypher stent. The strategy to implant a first stent proximally is unconventional, but is sometimes performed when treating a total occlusion with diffused disease in the distal part. Sometimes the first stenting implantation re-establishes a good flow and avoids the need to implant other stents more distally, or may just limit the total number of stents to be used. In this case, a second stent was implanted and this appeared sufficient. The small diagonal branch is treated with balloon angioplasty as shown in *frame 9*. The final result following implantation of two stents in the LAD is demonstrated in *frames 10* and *11*.

Message   The most important message of this case, besides stressing the value of the contra-lateral injection, is the fact that in some total occlusions with diffused distal disease, the implantation of stents occurs from proximal to distal rather than from distal to proximal; this is performed in order to better evaluate the distal vessel following good lumen establishment at the proximal level.

4. Parallel-wire technique for total occlusions

Case # 11272/03

This case (**Slides 1–5** (*frames 1–12*)) involves another example of occluded left anterior descending, performed on this occasion without contra-lateral injection. Baseline frames are shown in *frames 1* and *2*. Wire advancement in the mid-LAD was very complex and necessitated the use of the parallel-wire technique. The parallel-wire technique involves advancing a wire; if the first wire is not in the right lumen, this wire is left in place and the second wire is advanced parallel to the first wire in order to negotiate the true lumen. The advantage of leaving the first wire in place is to lead the operator to where the first lumen is located and where the second wire should not be directed. Finally, a wire is advanced in the distal LAD with true lumen negotiation (*frame 5*). The vessel is dilated with achievement of a fair angiographic result following angioplasty in *frame 8*. The combination of two different wires, Conquest Pro (Asahi Intec) and Dasher (Boston Scientific), contributed to this goal. The procedure is then completed with stent implantation. As usual with our approach to the treatment of total occlusions, and somewhat unconventionally, we proceeded from proximal to distal in order to better evaluate where to stop with stenting. We implanted a 33-mm-long proximal stent and then a second 33-mm Cypher stent. The final result appears adequate and is shown in *frames 11* and *12*.

Message The two elements illustrated in this case are the use of a parallel-wire technique with a stiff and soft wire (Conquest Pro and Dasher) and the usage of proximal-to-distal stent placement in total occlusions with diffuse distal disease.

5. Two total occlusions

Case # 11331/03

This case illustrates treatment of two total occlusions present in the same patient (**slides 1–7** (*frames 1–18*)). This occurrence is not so frequent, and what is even less frequent is the successful reopening of both total occlusions. The benefits in this particular case with a baseline left injection illustrated in *frames 1* and *2* is the presence of good contra-lateral collateralization as demonstrated in *frame 4*. The first lesion to be successfully crossed is the left anterior descending which was pre-dilated (*frame 6*) and a forward flow established in *frame 7*. Following implantation of two Cypher stents (33 mm long) the final result at the level of the LAD is demonstrated in *frame 10*. The circumflex was then effectively treated, with good results obtained following angioplasty at the level of a large and long obtuse marginal branch (*frame 13*). The procedure was completed with implantation of two long Cypher stents (33 mm), with achievement of an optimal result at the level of the circumflex and patency maintained at the level of the left anterior descending (*frames 14–16*). The large territory of distribution of the first obtuse marginal branch, which reaches the apex of the left ventricle, explains why the left anterior descending is of small diameter and short in its distal part. The final result in two projections is demonstrated in *frames 17* and *18*.

Message   This case illustrates that even the presence of two total occlusions at the proximal level in the left system is not a contra-indication to PCI procedure when the result can be consolidated with implantation of drug-eluting stents.

6. A technique of subintimal tracking to reopen a total occlusion: Case 1

Case HSR/SQI

This is a case (**slides 1–5** (*frames 1–12* and *run 1*)) of subtotal occlusion of the right coronary artery with total occlusion of the posterior descending. *Frames 1* and *2* illustrate the baseline lesion. The stenosis is crossed with a conventional soft wire, and POBA is performed with achievement of an acceptable result at the level of the proximal mid and distal right coronary artery to the postero-lateral branch. No posterior descending is visible. Following stent placement in the right coronary artery, a very faint stump is seen at the level of the posterior descending. This stump is illustrated in *frame 9*, and it may represent a dissection extending at the ostium of the posterior descending. In order to open this dissection towards the true lumen of the vessel, a technique of subintimal tracking and the entry is utilized. This technique takes advantage of the relatively atraumatic nature of a Whisper wire when a loop is created at the tip. The wire is gently advanced as shown in *run 1*, and a subintimal path is created until it reaches a more distal level and enters the true lumen (*frame 11*). *Frame 12* illustrates the posterior descending fully reopened with good reconstitution at the distal level. There is a dissection in the proximal part with good residual lumen and maintained flow. Sometimes these dissections need to be stented, but this decision depends on the evaluation of the residual lumen and on the distal flow. Recently, this technique of subintimal dissection has been utilized to open more proximal vessels, mainly right coronary artery, when a more conventional approach appears unsatisfactory.

Message   This case presents a new approach to reopen some very unfavorable chronic total occlusions.

7. A technique of subintimal tracking to reopen a total occlusion: Case 2

Case # 11875/04

This case (**slides 1–7** (*frames 1–19* and *run 1*)) illustrates treatment of a distal occlusion of the left anterior descending with the same new technique, which tries to advance with the creation of a subintimal track and then distal re-entry.

The baseline lesion is an occlusion of the mid LAD demonstrated in *frame 1*. Incidentally, there is also an occlusion of the circumflex and a focal stenosis of a large intermediate branch as demonstrated in *frames 1* and *2*.

First the operator treated the intermediate branch with a cutting balloon and Cypher-stent implantation, with a final good result as demonstrated in *frame 6*. Then an attempt was made to reopen the left anterior descending with different wires, and the final wire created a subintimal path with which it was difficult to progress more distally, as demonstrated in *frames 8, 9* and *10*. At that point, the wire (a Whisper wire) was used with a distal loop as shown in *frame 10* and then advanced in such a fashion as shown in *run 1*. This advancement extended the dissection with final re-entry at the level of the apex as demonstrated in *frame 11*. The left anterior descending was then reconstructed by implanting four long Cypher stents. There was an additional angioplasty on the diagonal branch. The final result is presented in *frames 14* and *15*. The LAD is well patent with preserved branches up to the apex, as demonstrated in the RAO projection inserted in *frame 15*. The procedure was then completed with treatment of the occlusion of the circumflex, which was relatively easily reopened and underwent implantation of a long Cypher stent.

Message   This case utilized the subintimal tracking technique with a re-entry, which can sometimes be the only approach to establish patency of a difficult chronic total occlusion (CTO).

8. Chronic total occlusion treatment with focal restenosis inside a Cypher: a different view according to angiography and IVUS

Case # 11082/02

This case (**slides 1–3** (*frames 1–8*)) illustrates treatment of in-stent restenosis, which presented with total occlusion of the left anterior descending. The occlusion dated more than 2 years and involves the left anterior descending following the origin of a large diagonal branch (*frame 1*). The stents implanted in the past were bare-metal stents. Following successful reopening of the occlusion, two Cypher stents were implanted with achievement of an excellent result. At 7-month follow-up, this case illustrates a rather typical and unique pattern of restenosis occurring when the Cypher stent fails. This pattern is a focal in-stent restenosis as demonstrated in *frame 6*. A unique finding is a dissociation between the clear evident image at the angiographic evaluation, as seen in *frame 7*, while the IVUS interrogation at the same site (*frame 8*) shows minimal or no tissue proliferation over the stent – definitely less than we would expect by examining the tight appearance of the angiogram. It is unclear why we see this dissociation, but this finding appears quite unique and infrequent when examining focal restenosis in Cypher stents.

Message   Some cases of focal restenosis in the Cypher stent may represent stent recoil or compression.

9. The Frontrunner device for chronic total occlusions

Case # 11147/02

This case (**slides 1, 2** (*frames 1–4*)) represents a total occlusion treated again with the help of contra-lateral injection from the left system. The baseline angiogram is shown in *frame 1* with no forward flow and no clear entering point. The device used to facilitate crossing of the occlusion is the Frontrunner (LuMend) catheter, which is a special spreading catheter utilized to treat total occlusions. The device is shown in the mid-right coronary artery in *frame 2*.

Following establishment of some sort of connection between the proximal and the distal lumen, a wire is successfully advanced in the distal right coronary artery and two long Cypher stents are implanted. Note that the nominal diameter of this stent is 3 mm, while the size of the artery is 3.5 mm. This situation was a drawback in the initial experience of Cypher stenting and forced the operator to over-dilate the 3-mm stent to 3.5 mm. It is a matter of debate whether this over-dilation affects the long-term result of drug-eluting stents.

Message   Even if not demonstrated, it is very reasonable always to use a 3.5-mm Cypher (seven-cell stent) in a 3.5-mm vessel rather than over-dilating a 3.0-mm Cypher (six-cell stent) to 3.5 mm or, even worse, to 4.0 mm.

10. Poor distal run-off after a full metal jacket for chronic total occlusion

Case # 11193/02

This case (**slides 1–3** (*frames 1–4* and *runs 1, 2*)) illustrates an unfavorable total occlusion of the right coronary artery in a patient post-coronary by-pass surgery. There are bridging collaterals from the mid to the most distal portion of the right coronary artery (*frame 1*). The device utilized in this procedure is the Frontrunner catheter, which is a spreading device advanced into the vessel without a guide wire. The procedure was complicated by extensive dissection involving the mid and distal part of the right coronary artery. There was some flow re-established into an acute marginal branch (*run 1*). Following wire manipulation, we were successful in regaining the distal lumen as demonstrated in *run 2*. The procedure was completed with implantation of four Cypher stents in the distal right coronary artery, acute marginal branch, and proximal right coronary artery. The final result appears adequate, even if there was some mismatching between the proximal part and the distal vessels as seen in the *run 2*. At the 5-month follow-up, unfortunately the right coronary artery appeared totally occluded. There were prominent collaterals from the left system. It is not clear how this event may have occurred, but it is conceivable that the large and sluggish flow in the proximal part of the artery with considerable foreign-body material, such as long stents, may compete unfavorably with the prominent and well-established collateralization from the left system.

Message   The message of this study is the need to evaluate carefully the final result in total occlusion before implanting several drug-eluting stents, which may occlude because of poor distal run-off.

11. Parallel-wire technique for chronic total occlusion

Case # 35956/04

This case is illustrated by **slides 1–4** (*frames 1–10*). *Frames 1* and *2* show a rather complex total occlusion with bridging collaterals involving the mid part of the right coronary artery.

The initial approach was to position an intermediate wire in the side branch, in order to better visualize and to maintain a better stability of the guiding catheter. We must acknowledge Dr Hideo Tamai who is the operator in this case. The first wire is advanced, but apparently not in the true lumen as demonstrated in *frame 5*. This brings into action the parallel-wire technique, developed by the members of the Japanese CTO club. This technique allows negotiation of two wires; ultimately one of the two wires will succeed in reaching the true lumen. Sometimes operators even utilized three wires in the same vessel. Following extensive manipulation, the operator was finally successful in reaching the distal lumen with a good preservation of the postero-lateral and PDA branches, as shown in *frame 8*. Following pre-dilatation, three Taxus stents were placed in this artery: two in the more distal branches and one proximal to the bifurcation. The final result is demonstrated in *frame 10*.

New approaches to chronic total occlusions

Kazuaki Mitsudo MD

PENETRATION STRATEGY USING CONQUEST PRO GUIDE-WIRE

Our approaches to the treatment of chronic total occlusions (CTO), and our penetration strategy with the use of the Conquest Pro guide-wire (Asahi Intec, Japan) are illustrated by slides 1–36.

Concept

When the guide-wire tip goes into the subintimal space, we can get the true lumen by using a steep and stiff-tip guide-wire and the landmark guide-wire method (seesaw wiring).

Equipment and devices

- Biplane cine machine (slide 19)
- Guide-catheter, 7- or 8-Fr
- Conquest Pro guide-wire(s) (slides 3–5)
- Over-the-wire support catheter(s) (slides 9–11)

Approach

- Transfemoral approach
- Bilateral puncture. Bilateral angiography
- Right femoral tandem puncture in case of occlusion of the left femoral artery
- Diagnostic catheter, 5- or 6-Fr, for contralateral injection

Guide-wire strategies and techniques

- Penetrating strategy instead of drilling strategy (Figure 1)
- Intermediate guide-wire to introduce the support catheter tip to the occlusion site
- Exchange the guide-wire for Conquest Pro (slides 3, 4)

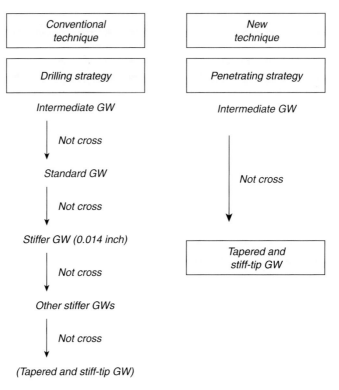

Figure 1   Drilling strategy and penetrating strategy. In conventional techniques, we formerly utilized numerous 0.014″ stiff guide-wires (GW) with drilling motion, which may cause larger subintimal space. We may call this technique the drilling strategy. However, we now use only the tapered-tip, highly stiff-tip guide-wire as a stiff wire, with less drilling motion. We call this the penetrating strategy

- Tip shape of Conquest Pro and the shaping device (slides 7, 8, Figure 2)
- Hint for using Conquest Pro guide-wire: Operator should gradually increase the force he uses to manipulate the wire, resulting in the same effects of stepwise exchange methods
- Seesaw wiring (slides 9–11, 14–16, Figures 3–5)

Angiographic and fluoroscopic strategy

The key to successful drilling and penetrating strategy:

- *Drilling strategy*: differentiating between true or false lumen by tactile response through the guidewire

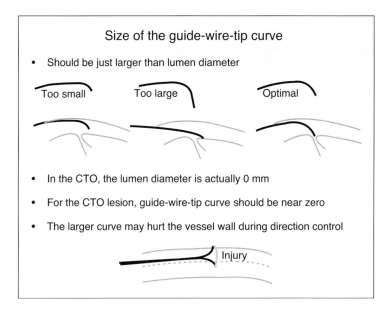

Figure 2   Optimal size of the guide-wire-tip curve in CTO lesions. In general, the size of the guide-wire-tip curve should be slightly larger than the lumen diameter for precise selection of the critical branch. In the CTO lesion, because the actual size of the lumen is estimated to be 0 mm, the curve size should be small, and if the curve of Conquest Pro is too large, the guide-wire tip may seriously damage the vessel wall during direction control

- *Penetrating strategy*: the tip direction of the guide-wire. The precise positioning and direction control of the guide-wire tip is much more important in the penetrating strategy
- *Before the procedure*: bilateral angiography to observe the detail around the occlusion site. Or time difference double dye injections in case of intracoronary collateral
- Biplane cine equipment. (Bidirectional angiography) (slides 19, 20)
- Projection angles perpendicular to the long axis of the vessel at region of interest (slide 18)

RESULTS

Single-center results are presented in slides 21–36. Historically, the main cause of failure of PCI for CTO was guide-wire failure, in which the guide-wire could not cross the lesion properly to the distal true lumen (slide 1). In turn, the main cause of guide-wire failure was the inability to make a re-entry from the sub-intimal space to the true lumen.

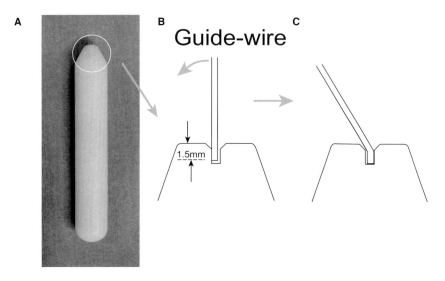

Figure 3 Shaping device of Conquest Pro's tip. A: Shaping device has a small pit, depth about 1.5 mm. To make a small tip-curve, the guide-wire tip is inserted in the small pit (B), and is angled to some degrees (C)

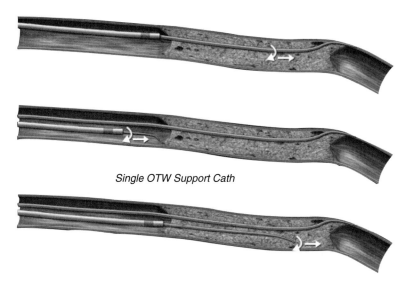

Figure 4 Parallel-wire method. The first guide-wire is used as a landmark, and the second one as a penetrating guide-wire. In the parallel-wire method, we use just one over-the-wire support catheter

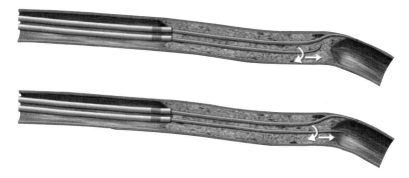

Figure 5 Seesaw wiring with double-support catheters. Seesaw wiring using two over-the-wire catheters at a time to perform the parallel-wire method can avoid the complex exchange procedure of over-the-wire catheter

A large subintimal space is inadequate for making a re-entry to true lumen (slide 2). It is easy to create a re-entry from a small subintimal lumen to a relatively large true lumen (slide 2, A). However, it is very difficult to make a re-entry from a large subintimal space to a relatively small true lumen (slide 2, B). Furthermore, in many failed cases, the enlarged subintimal space, or hematoma, pushes and makes the true lumen small. This makes creating re-entry from subintimal space to true lumen particularly difficult.

Examples of tapered and stiff-tip guide-wires are shown in slide 3. Among the Cross-IT XT family (Guidant), the Cross-IT XT 400 has the stiffest tip and is considered to be suitable for penetrating strategy. Conquest Pro has the most tapered and the stiffest tip.

The Conquest Pro guide-wire has a tapered tip from 0.014 to 0.009″ with 9 or 12 g stiffness with stainless-steel core wire and spring-coil structure (slide 4). It has an effective hydrophilic coating in the shaft, sparing the tip ball.

One of the advantages of the coating design of Conquest Pro is shown in slide 5. As shown in slide 6A, a high-lubricity tip makes it difficult for the guide-wire to catch the small dimple at the entry point, which can not be seen by angiography. As shown in slide 6B, a low-lubricity tip can more easily catch such a small dimple.

The optimal size of the guide-wire-tip curve in CTO lesions is described in slide 6. In general, the size of the guide-wire-tip curve should be slightly larger than the lumen diameter for precise selection of the critical branch. In the CTO lesion, because the actual size of the lumen is estimated at 0 mm, the curve size should be small. Furthermore if the curve of Conquest Pro is too large, the guide-wire tip may make a large injury in the vessel wall during direction control.

A tip curve of 1–2 mm is the smallest we can make in Conquest Pro (slide 7). The upper curve is for the initial penetration of entry point. If we fail to cross the lesion

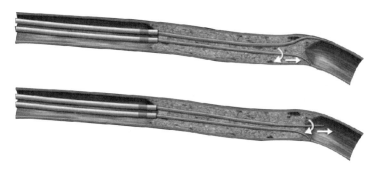

Figure 6   Seesaw wiring. We can change the role of each guide-wire very easily. If the second guide-wire can not find the true lumen, we can exchange the functions of two wires, that is, we can use the second wire as a landmark, and the first one as a penetrating one again

with the first shape of guide-wire tip, we use the more bent curve as shown in the lower part of the picture.

The shaping device of the Conquest Pro tip is shown in slide 8. As shown in slide 9A (Figure 3), the shaping device has a small pit, the depth of which is approximately 1.5 mm. To make a small tip curve, the guide-wire tip is inserted in the small pit (slide 9B), and is angled to several degrees (slide 9C).

The parallel-wire method is presented in slide 10 (Figure 4). The first guide-wire is used as a landmark, while the second is used as a penetrating guide-wire. In the parallel-wire method, we use just one over-the-wire support catheter.

Seesaw wiring is presented in slide 11 (Figure 5). Using two over-the-wire catheters at a time to perform the parallel-wire method, seesaw wiring can avoid the complex exchange procedure of the over-the-wire catheter. Seesaw wiring is considered further in slide 12 (Figure 6). We can change the role of each guide-wire very easily. If the second guide-wire can not get the true lumen, we can exchange the functions of the two wires. That is, we can use the second wire as a landmark, and the first one as a penetrating wire again.

Diagnostic CAG is presented in slide 13. Separate injection into LCA revealed the distal diagonal branch by bridge collateral. Slide 14 presents bilateral angiography in the same patient as in slide 13. Simultaneous bilateral coronary injections were made into both coronary arteries. Bilateral angiography revealed double CTOs in the LAD and diagonal branch (slide 14A) and after Y-stenting (slide 14B).

Slide 15 presents seesaw wiring and control angiography. A CTO lesion is revealed in the proximal RCA and bridge collaterals.

Slide 16 again presents seesaw wiring. The first Conquest Pro did not get the true lumen. Contra-lateral dye injection was used. (Slide 16A) RAO+CR; (slide 16B) LAO+CAU.

Slide 17 presents seesaw wiring. The second Conquest Pro got the true lumen. (Slide 17A) RAO+CR; (slide 17B) LAO+CAU.

Slide 18 presents seesaw wiring after stent implantation. (Slide 18A) RAO+CR; (slide 18B) LAO+CAU.

The following two points are key to a successful drilling and penetration strategy. For the drilling strategy, it is critical to differentiate, by tactile response of the guide-wire, the true or the false lumen. However, when using Conquest Pro, we can not feel the difference between the true and false lumen because of its tapered tip and lubricity. The precise positioning and direction control of the one guide-wire tip is much more important in the penetrating strategy. The best projection angles are perpendicular to the vessel axis at the region of interest. If the occlusion is long, as slide 19 shows, the suitable projection angles may be different according to the location of the guide-wire tip.

For the biplane or bidirectional angiography, the orthogonal projection angles have advantages over the other angles. As shown in slide 20, the sum of the blind area is smallest in the orthogonal projections. Blind area means that although the guide-wire is located in the subintimal space, it appears to be inside the true lumen. This leads to misperception, and orthogonal projections minimize this possibility.

As with slide 20, it is easier to get the true lumen by using the orthogonal projection angles as shown in slide 21. By the nonorthogonal projection angles (right part of the picture), the guide-wire risks going into the next blind area. If that occurs, it may be difficult to get the true lumen because of the large blind area. However, by using the orthogonal projections, there is less possibility of going into the blind area, leading to easier true lumen access.

We compared the results in *de novo* cases among four stages (slide 22). In stage one, we did not use the Conquest Pro guide-wire. In stage two, we used a conventional guide-wire exchange technique with the Conquest Pro guide-wire. In stage three, we implemented a new simple technique with the Conquest Pro guide-wire. In stage four, we performed a new simple technique with combination of Conquest Pro and the parallel-wire method or seesaw wiring.

The frequency of Conquest Pro guide-wire usage is shown in slide 23. Slide 24 (Figure 7) shows the overall guide-wire success rate.

The success rate with each vessel is shown in slide 25. The success rate was improved in all vessels – LAD, LCX and also RCA. In stage IV, the success rates were equivalent in all vessels.

As shown in slide 26, the success rate with long lesions is still low, but it improved significantly in stages III and IV.

In the lesion with an occlusion age dated more than 12 months, the improvement of success rate was most remarkable, as it also was for an occlusion of unknown age (slide 27).

As shown in slides 28 and 29, the success rates with heavily calcified lesions and with excessively tortuous lesions, respectively, are still low.

The multivariate analysis (slide 30, Table 1) shows that significant determinants of procedural failure are occlusion age, calcification, and long lesion in stages II and III.

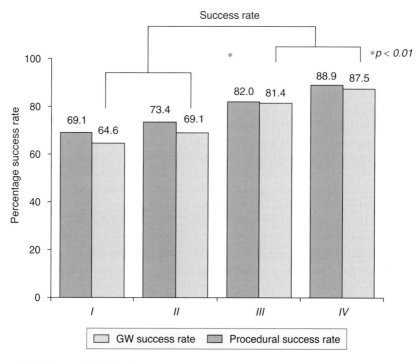

Figure 7   The overall guide-wire success rate

Table 1   Determinants of procedural failure in CTO. Multivariate analysis of procedural failure – Periods II and III

Variables	p-Value	Odds ratio (95% CI)
Occl. age (>3 months)	<0.001	3.15 (1.62–6.13)
Calcification	0.001	2.21 (1.37–3.57)
Long lesion	<0.001	1.96 (1.45–2.65)
Tortuosity	0.211	1.46 (0.81–2.65)
Side branch	0.645	1.09 (0.75–1.59)
Bridge collateral	0.647	1.10 (0.73–1.67)
Abrupt type	0.064	1.56 (0.98–2.50)

The multivariate analysis presented in **slide 31** (Table 2) shows that, in stage IV, tortuousity and calcification were significant determinants of procedural failure. Lesion length and occlusion age became insignificant. Tortous vessels and calcified lesions remain big problems with the penetrating strategy using Conquest Pro.

Table 2 Determinants of procedural failure in CTO. Multivariate analysis of procedural failure – Period IV

Variables	p-Value	Odds ratio (95% CI)
Tortuosity	<0.001	5.45 (2.05–14.51)
Calcification	0.003	3.64 (1.56–8.48)
Long lesion	0.091	1.92 (0.90–4.07)
Occl. age (> 3 months)	0.409	1.68 (0.49–5.79)
Side branch	0.572	0.78 (0.33–1.86)
Bridge collateral	0.089	0.41 (0.14–1.15)
Abrupt type	0.161	1.92 (0.77–4.80)

Table 3 Major complications

Period	I 95.1~96.9	II 96.10~98.10	III 98.11~01.3	IV 01.4~03.11	
No. of pts	165	241	201	271	p
AMI (%)	1.8	1.2	0.5	0.4	N.S.
Em CABG	0	0	0	0	
Death	0.6	0	0.5	0	
Tamponade	0.6	1.2	0.5	0.7	

Slide 32 shows that, for tortuous vessels, the additional gentle curve may be effective.

Slide 33 presents a tortuous occlusion with bridge collaterals. (Slide 33A) LAO+cranial; (slide 33B) RAO+caudal. Slide 34 shows the same case, with seesaw wiring and the curve for the tortuous vessel. The first Conquest guide-wire went into the subintimal space. (The proximal guide-wire was Whisper guide-wire). (Slide 34A) LAO+cranial; (slide 34B) RAO+caudal; (slide 34C) the curve shown in slide 32.

Slide 35 shows the same case as in slide 33, with seesaw wiring. The second Conquest Pro achieved the distal true lumen. Slide 36 also shows the same case as in slide 33, after stent implantation.

As shown in slide 37 (Table 3), the incidence of tamponade was not higher in the Conquest era.

CONCLUSIONS

In conclusion, the new technique of PCI for CTO using the Conquest Pro guide-wire and seesaw wiring is simple, safe and has a very high initial success rate. This technique could become one of the standards.

COMPLEX LESIONS
PART VI – THROMBUS-CONTAINING LESIONS

Approach to thrombus-containing lesions

Issam Moussa MD

Case 1

Case 1 is an example of a small thrombus-causing embolization after percutaneous transluminal coronary angioplasty (PTCA) in native coronary artery **(slides 1–3)**.

Clinical presentation

A 63-year-old patient presented with acute coronary syndrome.

Coronary angiography and intervention

- **Slide 1 (a)**. Baseline coronary angiography (RAO view) illustrates a proximal LCX artery thrombotic lesion (arrow)
- **Slide 2 (b)**. The lesion was pre-dilated with a Maverick II balloon (2.5×15 mm) inflated at 8 atm
- **Slide 2 (c)**. Coronary angiography after pre-dilatation demonstrates delayed flow and a new angiographic cutoff (embolus) of the distal LCX artery (arrow)
- **Slide 3 (d)**. A Cypher stent (3.0×13 mm) was deployed at 16 atm
- **Slide 3 (e)**. Final coronary angiography demonstrates good stent deployment, but persistent delayed coronary flow and a distal LCX embolus

Educational points

- Occurrence of slow flow and distal embolization with native coronary thrombotic lesions is unpredictable. Even a small thrombus can lead to distal embolization and slow flow

- Slow flow and distal embolization can still occur despite optimal antithrombotic and antiplatelet therapy

Measures to reduce the likelihood of slow flow and distal embolization (thrombectomy, distal protection devices) should be considered in these patients.

Case 2

Case 2 (slides 1–6) presents an example showing treatment of the native coronary artery with a large thrombus burden using the Possis Angiojet device and the PercuSurge Guardwire (Medtronic) without percutaneous transluminal coronary angioplasty (PTCA) and stenting.

Clinical presentation

A 73-year-old patient presented within 24 h after inferior wall myocardial infarction.

Coronary angiography and intervention

- Slide 1 (a). Baseline coronary angiography (LAO view) illustrates a proximal thrombotic RCA occlusion (arrow)
- Slide 2 (b). Coronary angiography after wire introduction illustrates a very large thrombus, extending from proximal to distal RCA with aneurysmal dilatation
- Slide 3 (c). Hydrolytic thrombectomy with the Possis Angiojet device was performed in conjunction with distal protection using the PercuSurge Guardwire (Medtronic)
- Slide 4 (d). Coronary angiography after hydrolytic thrombectomy demonstrates significant reduction in thrombus burden, but with abrupt angiographic cutoff of the PLS branch
- Slide 5 (e). The PLS branch was wired and Nipride was infused through an Ultra Fuse X catheter (Boston Scientific)
- Slide 6 (f). Final coronary angiography demonstrates patent RCA with TIMI III flow

Educational points

- The presence of a very large subacute thrombus burden, such as in this case, makes it extremely unlikely that balloon angioplasty and stenting alone can achieve acceptable arterial patency with TIMI III flow
- The use of thrombectomy alone is plausible, but still carries the risk of distal embolization. The use of large-profile filter-based distal protection devices may cause distal embolization through the delivery stage. The use of balloon-based distal protection may be effective, but frequently the export catheter tip becomes occluded when such a large thrombus burden is present

- This case illustrates a typical setting, where a combination of thrombectomy and distal protection can be helpful

Case 3

Case 3 (slides 1–10) is an example of treating bifurcational thrombotic lesions with a combination of thrombectomy, distal protection, and the crush technique.

Clinical presentation

Case 3 involved a 70-year-old patient in whom thrombolytic therapy for anterior-wall myocardial infarction had not been successful.

Coronary angiography and intervention

- **Slide 1 (a)**. Baseline RAO and LAO cranial angiographic view illustrates a proximal LAD thrombotic sub-occlusion (TIMI I flow) involving the ostium of the 1st diagonal branch (TIMI I flow)
- **Slide 2 (b)**. A PercuSurge Guard-wire was used to cannulate the LAD artery, and a short BMW Universal wire (Guidant) was used to cannulate the diagonal branch. Hydrolytic thrombectomy using the Possis Angiojet was performed with distal protection
- **Slide 3 (c)**. Coronary angiography after hydrolytic thrombectomy demonstrates significantly reduced thrombus burden and TIMI III flow in the LAD and diagonal branch
- **Slide 4 (d)**. The ostium of the 1st diagonal branch was dilated with a Maverick II balloon (2.5 × 15 mm)
- **Slide 4 (e)**. Coronary angiography was performed after balloon dilatation of the diagonal branch
- **Slides 5–8 (f-1 to f-4)**. Two Cypher stents were deployed in the LAD (3.0 × 23 mm) and diagonal branch (3.0 × 18 mm) using the crush technique. Post-dilatation was performed with a Quantum Maverick balloon (Boston Scientific) (3.5 × 15 mm) in the LAD and a Quantum Maverick balloon (2.5 × 15 mm) in the diagonal branch using kissing inflation
- **Slides 9 and 10 (g-1 to g-2)**. Final coronary angiography demonstrates widely patent stents without any evidence of distal embolization and TIMI III flow

Educational points

The approach to thrombus-laden bifurcation lesions presents several challenges:

- A simple approach using balloon dilatation to both the LAD and diagonal branch increases the likelihood of distal embolization to one or both territories

- An attempt to use balloon dilatation with distal protection in only one territory does not eliminate the risk of embolization to the other unprotected territory
- One of two approaches can be used to minimize the risk of embolization:
  - Employ simultaneous distal protection in both branches
  - We chose to perform thrombectomy with distal protection in the main vessel to remove the thrombus from the bifurcation. This reduces the risk of embolization to the side branch during balloon angioplasty
- After thrombus removal, we proceeded with bifurcation stenting using the crush technique. Owing to severe ostial branch disease, which reduces the chances of success with balloon angioplasty alone, provisional stenting was not attempted

Case 4

Case 4 (slides 1–13) is an example of treating bifurcational thrombotic lesions with a combination of thrombectomy, distal protection, and the crush technique.

Clinical presentation

A 53-year-old patient presented 24 h after sustaining anterior wall myocardial infarction.

Coronary angiography and intervention

- **Slide 1 (a)**. The baseline coronary angiography (RAO cranial view) illustrates a proximal LAD thrombotic occlusive lesion involving the 1st diagonal branch (TIMI 0 flow)
- **Slide 2 (b)**. Both the LAD and the diagonal branch were wired. Hydrolytic thrombectomy with the Posiss Angiojet device was performed towards the LAD
- **Slide 3 (c)**. Coronary angiography after hydrolytic thrombectomy demonstrates reduced thrombus burden in the LAD with improved TIMI flow in both the LAD and the diagonal branch. However, note the large thrombus burden in the diagonal branch (arrow)
- **Slide 4 (d)**. Hydrolytic thrombectomy was performed in the diagonal branch
- **Slide 5 (e)**. Coronary angiography after hydrolytic thrombectomy in the diagonal branch demonstrates no significant change in thrombus burden
- **Slide 6 (f)**. An EPI filter wire was positioned in the distal segment of the diagonal branch and balloon angioplasty was performed (Maverick II balloon, 3.0×20 mm, at 16 atm)
- **Slide 7 (g)**. Coronary angiography after PTCA with distal protection in the diagonal branch. Note the reduction in thrombus burden and improved flow. However, there remain severe stenoses in the LAD and the ostium of the diagonal branch

- **Slide 8 (h).** Coronary angiography after cutting balloon angioplasty for the LAD and the ostium of the diagonal branch
- **Slides 9–11 (i-1 to i-3).** Two Cypher stents were deployed in the LAD (3.5×18 mm) and ostial diagonal branch (3.0×18 mm) using the crush technique
- **Slides 12–13 (j-1 to j-2).** Final coronary angiography demonstrates widely patent stents and TIMI III flow in both territories

Educational points

- In this case, the use of hydrolytic thrombectomy yielded discrepant results in the same patient. There was noticeable reduction in thrombus burden in the LAD, but no reduction of thrombus burden in the diagonal branch
- This case illustrates that the use of filter-based distal protection in native coronary thrombotic lesions is feasible and can be effective in reducing embolization

Case 5

Case 5 (slides 1–9) is an example of treating a Cypher-stent thrombosis with thrombectomy, cutting balloon, and distal protection.

Clinical presentation

A 55-year-old patient presented with subacute stent thrombosis 8 days post-Cypher-stent implantation.

Coronary angiography and intervention

- **Slide 1 (a).** Baseline RAO cranial angiographic view illustrates the original lesions treated (90% diffuse proximal LAD lesion involving the 1st diagonal branch). Note that the mid-LAD is occluded
- **Slide 2 (b).** A final RAO cranial angiographic view after deployment of a Cypher stent (3.0×33 mm) extending into the diagonal branch. (Note the residual distal disease in the diagonal branch)
- **Slide 3 (c).** Coronary angiography in the RAO cranial view 8 days after the original procedure was performed after the patient presented with an acute ST elevation myocardial infarction (note the stent occlusion)
- **Slide 4 (d).** Coronary angiography after stent recanalization using a PT2 moderate wire in an over-the-wire balloon (note the thrombus in the stent)
- **Slide 5 (e).** A PercuSurge Guardwire (arrow) was introduced, and a Cypher stent (2.5×8 mm) was deployed to cover the lesion distal to the original stent (arrow)

- Slide 6 (f). Hydrolytic thrombectomy using the Possis Angiojet device (arrow) with distal protection using the PercuSurge Guardwire (arrow)
- Slide 7 (g). Coronary angiography after hydrolytic thrombectomy demonstrating significantly reduced thrombus burden, but with a small residual filling defect (arrow)
- Slide 8 (h). Cutting balloon angioplasty performed at the site of the filling defect with distal protection followed by aspiration
- Slide 9 (i). Final coronary angiography demonstrates fully patent stent with TIMI III flow

Educational points

- This case illustrates that the techniques of thrombectomy, distal protection, and cutting balloon should not be viewed as being competitive, but as being synergistic devices that may serve different purposes in a given clinical scenario

Case 6

Case 6 (slides 1–11) is an example of treating subtotal tortuous RCA with drug-eluting stents, with an emphasis on wire access and stent deliverability issues.

Clinical presentation

A 69-year-old patient presented with unstable angina.

Coronary angiography and intervention

- Slides 1 and 2 (a-1 to a-2). Baseline LAO and RAO coronary angiography illustrates 95% proximal and distal RCA lesions with severe tortuousity. The guide-catheter shown is a 6-Fr-AL1 guide with side holes
- Slides 3 and 4 (b-1 to b-2). LAO coronary angiogram with (1) and without (2) contrast showing a 0.0014″ Dasher wire (Boston Scientific, or Target Therapeutics) inside a Transit catheter (Cordis) (arrow), with the tip of the wire just proximal to the distal lesion
- Slide 5 (c). The Dasher wire was not able to traverse the distal lesion, so it was replaced with a PT2 Intermediate wire that traversed the distal lesion. However, the wire could not be advanced further owing to inadequate guide support. An attempt to engage the guide further led to guide disengagement
- Slide 6 (d). The 6-Fr AL1 guide-catheter was replaced with a 7-Fr MP guide-catheter with side holes. Subsequently, we were able to cannulate the RCA using a Dasher wire with the Transit catheter support. The Dasher wire was then replaced with a BMW Universal wire (note the extent of pseudo-stenoses as a result of artery straightening)

- **Slide 7 (e)**. An LAO coronary angiogram after pre-dilatation of the proximal and distal RCA lesions with a Maverick II (2.5×20-mm) balloon
- **Slide 8 (f)**. An attempt to deliver a Cypher stent (2.5×23 mm) to the distal RCA lesion failed. Subsequently, a Taxus stent (2.5×20 mm) was successfully delivered
- **Slide 8 (g)**. Coronary angiography (LAO view) after Taxus stent deployment for the distal lesion (note the lumen compromise at the proximal edge-arrow head)
- **Slide 9 (h)**. An attempt to deliver the Cypher stent (2.5×23 mm) to cover the mid-RCA lesion also failed. This stent was deployed in the proximal RCA
- **Slide 9 (i)**. Coronary angiography (LAO view) after deployment of the Cypher stent at the proximal lesion (note the residual mid-RCA disease)
- **Slide 10 (j)**. A Taxus stent (3.0×28 mm) was successfully delivered to the mid-RCA lesion through the Cypher stent and deployed successfully
- **Slides 10 and 11 (k-1 to k-2)**. LAO and RAO coronary angiography shows the final result

Educational points

Catheter-based coronary intervention in severely tortuous coronary anatomy still presents several challenges:

- Guide-catheter support remains a critical component of the decision-making process. The choice of the guiding catheter should be individualized to the specific anatomy. Despite the fact that an AL1 catheter provides excellent support in RCA interventions, it was not the ideal guide in the current case
- In tortuous anatomy, tapered and hydrophilic wires facilitate arterial cannulation. When using hydrophilic wires, however, care should be taken to avoid subintimal passage, particularly at curved segments
- The use of an over-the-wire end-hole catheter provides a vehicle for wire support and exchange. However, this catheter should be kink-resistant
- Stent deliverability is of paramount importance. In this particular case, the Taxus stent clearly out-performed the Cypher stent

4
Surgical Arena

Left main stenting

1. Crush or V-technique for a short left main with bifurcational disease

Case # 10974/02

Case # 10974/02 is illustrated by **slides 1–5** (*frames 1–12*). *Frames 1* and *2* show a moderate disease of the left main, extending into the proximal left anterior descending (LAD) with severe ostial disease of the circumflex. This particular anatomy demands stenting for both branches. The technical approach in this situation varies according to the experience of the operator. This relatively short left main is potentially suitable for V-stenting. In this particular case, we elected to use the crush technique. *Frame 3* demonstrates both stents in place, while *frame 4* demonstrates final kissing inflation. This case represents one of our early experiences with the crush technique, and the procedure was not preceded by aggressive cutting balloon pre-dilatation, particularly of the ostium of the circumflex. *Frames 5–7* show deployment of an additional stent at the ostium of the left main, while *frame 8* shows the final result. Despite the lack of what we call 'optimal lesion preparation', we were rewarded by a good follow-up result with absence of any recurrence, as demonstrated in the 9-month follow-up (*frames 9–12*).

Message   If we choose the V-technique, we have to leave the new carina reasonably proximally into the left main. At present, we do not know the long-term outcome of leaving this double stent layer in a vessel when utilizing drug-eluting stents. In case a proximal stent needs to be implanted, it is almost always worth taking the risk of leaving a small gap, and the stent needs to be directed towards one of the two arms of the V.

2. Unprotected left main bifurcational stenting with cutting balloon pre-dilatation

Case # 11728/03

This is another example (**slides 1–4** (*frames 1–11*)) of unprotected left main stenting with long lesions involving the circumflex branch. *Frames 1* and *2* illustrate the baseline angiography.

As, most of the time, we favor pre-dilatation of both branches, we pre-dilated the circumflex with a cutting balloon 6 mm long (*frame 3*). *Frame 4* is important, because in addition to showing the pre-dilatation of the left anterior descending, it shows that we have a balloon pump in place, which is a common setting in this type of procedure. *Frame 5* shows the result following pre-dilatation.

Frames 6 and *7* show the different steps of the crush technique, which allowed coverage also of a more distal lesion in the circumflex. As usual, the first inflated stent is the one in the circumflex (*frame 7*) then, following removal of the stent and of the wire from that branch, the stent in the LDA is inflated (*frame 8*). The final kissing is demonstrated in *frame 9*. *Frames 10* and *11* show the final result in both projections.

Message   The main message in this case, as in many of the others, is that in complex bifurcations involving large territories, it is crucial to guarantee the opening of both branches at a very early stage, avoiding the risk of not being able to stent one of the two branches. For this reason, the V-technique or the crush technique are, in our view, the most simple approach to this type of anatomy.

3. Directional atherectomy of the main branch to obtain access to the side branch

Case # 11717/03

Case # 11717/03 is illustrated by **slides 1–5** (*frames 1–13*). *Frames 1* and *2* show the baseline angiogram of this lesion involving the distal segment of the left main, with a sharp angulation of the circumflex artery. The left anterior descending is protected by a functioning mammary artery. The first approach was to try to wire both the diagonal branch coming off the proximal LAD and the circumflex. Owing to the sharp angulation of the circumflex, we were not able to negotiate the wire at this level, despite numerous attempts. We used several wires, including Pilot (Guidant) and Dasher (Target Therapeutics). For this reason, we selected to perform directional atherectomy in the LAD (*frame 3*). With this maneuver, we felt that some debulking would have allowed an easier passage of the wire into the circumflex. The result following atherectomy is shown in *frame 4*. Following this procedure, we were able to advance the wire into the circumflex (*frame 5*), and then we dilated both vessels (for the circumflex we used the cutting balloon). *Frame 7* shows the result following cutting balloon dilatation. We believe that the approach of performing atherectomy to negotiate a wire into a branch when the anatomy is not favorable is unusual, and it is one of the first case in which we have used it. Theoretically, plaque removal in the main branch may facilitate entrance into the side branch, as demonstrated in this case. Following this maneuver, we proceeded to position the stent into the intermediate branch and the LAD with the crush technique, as demonstrated in *frames 8–10*. The final kissing inflation, as usual, is performed at the end of the procedure, as shown in *frame 11*. The final result with preservation of all three major branches is demonstrated in *frames 12* and *13*.

Message   The main message of this case, besides the usual one regarding utilization of the crush technique in order to maintain patency of multiple branches at the same time, is the utilization of a debulking technique to gain wire access into a side branch, which before debulking could not be accessed.

4. A high-risk left main lesion

Case # 10971/02

This is an example (**slides 1–4** (*frames 1–11*)) of a high-risk unprotected left main lesion, in an elderly patient with a low ejection fraction and diffuse disease of the left anterior descending and with occluded right coronary artery. Owing to poor general conditions, this patient was not considered suitable for surgical revascularization, and a percutaneous revascularization was performed. As *frames 1* and *2* demonstrate, there is severe narrowing in the distal left main and diffuse disease in the proximal and mid left anterior descending. The procedure was performed with intra-aortic balloon counter-pulsation (*frame 3*). Both vessels (LAD and circumflex) were wired, and the left main was pre-dilated towards the circumflex (*frame 4*). Following that procedure, the LAD was pre-dilated and we implanted a long Cypher stent (*frame 6*). The next step was to treat the left main. In order to assure immediate patency of both vessels (LAD and circumflex), the crush technique was selected. *Frame 8* shows inflation of the stent into the circumflex, while another stent is in position from the left main towards the LAD. The next step (*frame 9*) is deployment of the stent in the LAD. There is no question that this approach is the one that will give immediate patency of both arteries (as with the V-technique). The risk is minimal at the time of recrossing into one branch because patency of the branch is provided by the presence of a stent. In general, we always try to perform kissing balloon inflation. In our experience, the initial cases in which we could not or we did not perform kissing-balloon inflations were not associated with a risk of thrombosis. We suspect that the lack of this final maneuver may not optimize the protection against restenosis. *Frames 10* and *11* show the final result. This particular patient had a good short-term clinical outcome. However, 5 weeks after the procedure, antiplatelet therapy was fully stopped due to an intercurrent disease, and the patient sustained fatal thrombosis of the stents.

Message   This particular situation stresses the current limitation of drug-eluting stents for unprotected left main treatment: the patient is fully dependent on antiplatelet therapy, and any risk associated with stopping antiplatelet therapy may translate into the risk of death. These decisions are important when evaluating patient for possible unprotected left main stenting.

5. The risks of the 'culottes' technique in left main trunk

Case # 11583/03

This is a patient who had left mammary implantation on the left anterior descending with graft failure and came to our attention for angioplasty on this unprotected left main coronary artery (**slides 1–6** (*frames 1–12*)). The lesion was attempted with the intent to perform a culotte technique. Due to the relatively favorable angulations and the size of the vessels, we elected to perform this procedure without balloon pump support. *Frames 1–3* show a baseline anatomy. Following wiring of both branches, the circumflex was pre-dilated and a Taxus stent was positioned in this vessel. The LAD was then rewired, and dilatation of the struts towards this vessel was performed without difficulties. At that point, a second Taxus stent was advanced towards the LAD. There were problems in crossing towards the LAD, and during these attempts the vessel abruptly closed and the patient had hemodynamic collapse (*frame 6*). A Zeta stent (Guidant) was successfully advanced into the LAD, reestablishing flow in this vessel. In addition, balloon counterpulsation was initiated. Following stabilization, the procedure was completed with implantation of a short Taxus stent from the left main towards the left anterior descending (*frame 8*). The stent was then crossed and dilated towards the circumflex (*frame 9*), and final kissing balloon inflation was performed (*frame 10*). The final result was good (*frames 11* and *12*).

Message   This case illustrates the potential problems of performing the culottes technique, associated with the fact that we always need to remove the wire from one of the two branches.

Particularly in situations of unprotected left main stenting, this technique should be performed, in our view, with intra-aortic balloon counter-pulsation support. Overall, we are not sure whether the complexity and the added risk of the culottes technique are counter-balanced by a significant low restenosis rate when utilizing drug-eluting stents. For all these reasons, we now prefer to use the crush technique, which allows immediate patency of both vessels, in high-risk lesions.

6. Restenosis in a DES implanted on a left main coronary artery

Case # 10845/02

This is an interesting case (**slides 1–5** (*frames 1–12*)) of recurrent restenosis despite drug-eluting stent implantation.

Frames 1 and *2* show the baseline lesion in the distal left main, with the other vessels relatively preserved. The original lesion was treated initially with a Cypher-stent implantation (six cells 3 mm in diameter). Owing to the large size of the left main, the stent was post-dilated with a 3.5-mm balloon (*frame 3*). At the 6-month follow-up, the angiogram showed focal restenosis in the mid of the left main (*frame 4*). This time, the operator decided to re-treat this restenosis with a new angioplasty and without additional stenting, with a good final result (*frame 10*).

Unfortunately, at follow-up, there was a second restenosis which involved the proximal LAD and the body of the left main, and with occlusion of the circumflex.

This case also represents the rare but possible event of diffuse or even total occlusion of the vessel treated with drug-eluting stents.

Message   Our current practice is to almost always treat in-stent restenosis occurring inside a drug-eluting stent with implantation of another drug-eluting stent. Sometimes we use the same type (Cypher on Cypher); at other times, we may use a different type (Taxus on a Cypher). We have no specific rule by which to make a particular choice. The reason why we use another drug-eluting stent is because we assume that the lesion which has failed a drug-eluting stent one time is particularly aggressive, and we cannot afford to fail a second time. There are cases of a second restenosis in a drug-eluting stent in which we successfully implanted two drug-eluting stents (one on top of each other) during the same procedure (sandwich technique). Follow-up of these cases has been very favorable without any further recurrence.

Multivessel treatment

1. Complex multivessel disease with good follow-up result

Case # 11021/02

This is a typical example (**slides 1–3** (*frames 1–7*)) of a very diffuse disease involving three arteries treated with multiple stent implantations with excellent immediate results and, more importantly, results maintained at follow-up. *Frames 1* and *2* show multiple lesions in the obtuse marginal branch, left anterior descending, and right coronary artery. The approach of covering fully a lesion with various stents was taken by placing first one long stent in the obtuse marginal branch and then four long stents in the left anterior descending. The right coronary artery was treated with three stents. These steps are illustrated in *frames 3–5* (the final result after stent implantation). More importantly, preserved optimal vessel patency at the angiographic follow-up at 10 months is presented in *frames 6* and *7*. The branches are all patent, with minimal neointimal hyperplasia.

We believe that this approach would have been totally impossible and very difficult to conceive in the era of bare-metal stents.

2. Multiple stents for diffuse disease

Case # 10941/02

This is an example (**slides 1–5** (*frames 1–15*)) of diffuse disease involving the left anterior descending and more focal lesions at the level of the circumflex (obtuse marginal branch) and right coronary artery.

The baseline anatomy is shown in *frames 1–3*. The LAD was treated with seven Cypher stents, utilizing the crush technique at the level of the bifurcation of the diagonal branch. The obtuse marginal branch and the right coronary artery were treated in a more focal fashion owing to the presence of rather short lesions. The most gratifying element is the fact that the angiographic follow-up performed at 10 months demonstrated only the presence of a focal restenosis, very short in length, in the mid segment of the LAD. It is important to mention that the exercise test, including thallium scintigraphy performed 1 week prior to the angiographic follow-up, was completely negative, and the patient was fully asymptomatic despite vigorous physical exercise. As in other cases, this approach illustrates how durable the result can be despite utilizing a 'full metal jacket' approach, which was frequently associated with diffuse restenosis in the past. In this specific case, despite the absence of demonstrable ischemia, the operator felt that it was appropriate to correct this focal restenosis with cutting balloon inflations, as shown in *frames 10–12*; a good final result was achieved, as demonstrated in *frame 15*.

Frame 12 is also interesting because it demonstrates the long-term follow-up of a 2.25×18 mm stent at the apical LAD, which maintained good patency with minimal or absent hyperplasia.

Message   With drug-eluting stents, it is important to cover completely the diseased segment, even if this task sometimes may require many stents, particularly if we consider our prior experience with bare-metal stents.

3. Complex multivessel disease treatment

Case # 11443/03

This case is another example (**slides 1–22** (*frames 1–52*)) of diffuse multivessel disease, with a total occlusion of the mid circumflex and double complex bifurcational lesions of the diagonal branch and of the left anterior descending, in a patient with diabetes mellitus.

The baseline angiogram is shown in *frames 1* and *2*. The first vessel to be treated was the circumflex as shown in *frames 3–5*. Following lesion pre-dilatation, including cutting balloon at the level of the bifurcation (*frames 6* and *7*), Taxus stents were deployed with the crush technique (*frames 9–11*). The final result was completed with another stent placed more proximally in the circumflex, and post-dilatation with a larger balloon at high pressure at the level of the proximal circumflex (*frame 14*). The final result at the level of the circumflex appears excellent, as demonstrated in *frames 15* and *16*.

The next vessel to be treated was the double bifurcation at the level of the diffusely diseased LAD and diagonal branch (*frame 18*). Wiring at the level of the three branches was performed, and pre-dilatation at each level was accomplished. We may add that today, in this diffusely diseased vessel, we would also employ the cutting balloon to achieve better pre-dilatation. Crushing stenting was performed inside the secondary bifurcation of the diagonal branch, trying not to protrude into the left anterior descending. This is demonstrated in *frames 23* and *24*. Following this maneuver and after post-dilatation at the level of the main branch of the diagonal, a kissing inflation at this level was performed utilizing a fixed-wire Ace balloon (Boston Scientific) (*frames 27* and *28*).

The next vessel to be treated was the left anterior descending. *Frame 29* shows the result at the bifurcation of the diagonal branch following kissing inflation. Following pre-dilatation of the left anterior descending, including cutting balloon at proximal distal, and mid-level (*frames 33* and *34*), the vessel appears diffusely dissected but well dilated. (Please note a large septal branch in *frame 35*.) The next treatment involved multiple Cypher stents implanted distally, mid, and proximally. The very proximal stent in *frame 39* is a Taxus stent because a Cypher stent could not be negotiated at this level, despite the fact that the other Cypher stents were able to be advanced. The result after dilatation with a crush technique of the proximal bifurcation in the left anterior descending, including kissing balloon inflation, is shown in *frames 43* and *44*. The final optimal result is seen except for a possible persistent compromise of the ostium of the left anterior descending, as shown in *frame 43*. This finding prompted performance of a 'reverse' crush at this level, with implantation of an additional short Cypher stent and a Powersail balloon (Guidant) post-dilatation to crush the protruding part of the stent into the proximal LAD, with the Powersail positioned towards the diagonal branch. The final result is shown in *frame 48*.

The 6-month follow-up shows a persistent patency at the level of the left anterior descending and diagonal branches (*frames 49* and *50*), with an occlusion of the circumflex. Because there was no associated acute clinical event, we define this late occlusion of the circumflex as aggressive restenosis, rather than thrombosis. *Frames 51* and *52* show the immediate result at the level of the circumflex and the follow-up. The other difference between the circumflex and the left anterior descending was the fact that in the former vessel the Taxus stents were used, while in the second vessel the Cypher stents were used – except for the very proximal stent which was the Taxus. It is also worth noticing that the large septal branch seen in *frame 35* and occluded during the procedure (see *frame 40*) turned out to be patent (*frame 49*) at follow-up.

Message   This very complex and time-consuming case tells us that, with appropriate dedication, a full vessel reconstruction can be achieved well.

It is not easy to understand why the circumflex artery closed despite an excellent immediate result. It is possible then that low distal run-off could have contributed to this event.

4. Multivessel disease: do we really need to debulk before implanting DES? Searching for a single-digit TVR in multivessel stenting

Case # 10943/02

This is another example (**slides 1–8** (*frames 1–18*)) of triple-vessel disease involving the LAD, the obtuse marginal branch, and total occlusion of the right coronary artery.

Baseline anatomy is shown in *frames 1* and *2*. Note the sub-occluded obtuse marginal branch and collateral circulation through the occluded right coronary artery. The right coronary artery is seen in *frame 4*. The first step was reopening of the right coronary artery with implantation of three long Cypher stents, as shown in *frame 6*. *Frame 8* demonstrates achievement of an optimal final result.

The next step was to open the obtuse marginal branch and perform debulking of this diffusely diseased vessel with the Silverhawk (Foxhollow) atherectomy catheter, as shown in *frame 10*. The result was completed with positioning of a long Cypher stent at this level. *Frame 13* demonstrates the final result at the level of the obtuse marginal branch. Atherectomy was then continued in the LAD up to the bifurcation, and a Cypher stent was positioned in the LAD without any stent at the level of the diagonal branch. The final result is presented in *frames 17* and *18*.

Message   This case illustrates the possibility of combining atherectomy and Cypher or other drug-eluting stent implantation. At the present time, there are no specific guidelines concerning the use of debulking with drug-eluting stents. Our personal view is that in medium-to-small vessels presenting with diffuse disease involving long segments, the combination of these two techniques (debulking and drug-eluting stents) may be of value. Unfortunately, there is a lack of dedicated studies on this operator-dependent condition.

5. Complete revascularization utilizing Taxus and Cypher stents

Case # 11714/02

This case is another example of multivessel disease treated with complete revascularization using drug-eluting stents (slides 1–8 (*frames 1–19*)). The baseline angiogram is shown in *frames 1* and *2*. There is diffuse disease of the large intermediate branch, multiple lesions in the left anterior descending coronary artery (LAD), and multiple lesions in the circumflex and the right coronary artery (as shown in *frames 3* and *4*).

The first vessel to be treated with three long stents is the right coronary artery as shown in *frame 6*, with the final result presented in *frames 7* and *8*. The intermediate branch is then pre-dilated utilizing the cutting balloon at various levels, as shown in *frame 10*. It is our approach to utilize the cutting balloon in medium-to-small vessels with diffuse disease. The vessel is then treated with two long Cypher stents, with the final result demonstrated in *frame 13*. The next step involves treatment of the left anterior descending with two long Taxus stents as shown in *frames 15* and *16*. The very proximal lesion in the left anterior descending is then treated with a large Taxus stent as shown in *frame 18*. The final result is presented in *frame 19*.

6. Combination of debulking and stenting in a patient considered to be at very high risk of restenosis

Case # 11578/03

This case is another example (slides 1–11 (*frames 1–25*)) of triple-vessel disease with medium-size vessels and diffuse disease. These lesions were treated by combining atherectomy and stenting. The baseline images of the left coronary artery are shown in *frames 1* and *2*. The first step was to perform IVUS-guided atherectomy at the level of the circumflex, utilizing the Silverhawk catheter (Foxhollow). When dealing with a small vessel with diffused disease, the confidence to perform atherectomy, particularly at the distal level, is present only following confirmation by IVUS that the vessel is of appropriate size for this technology. The result was completed with implantation of two long Cypher stents as shown in *frames 6* and *7. Frame 9* shows the final results at the level of the obtuse marginal branch.

The procedure was then continued at the level of the left anterior descending.

Again IVUS guidance gave reassurance that the vessel was of appropriate size to be treated with this technology. The result is completed with the implantation of two long Taxus stents at the level of the left anterior descending. DCA was then performed at the level of the medium-to-small diagonal branch, and a long Taxus stent was implanted at this level (*frame 18*). The final result without coverage of the bifurcation LAD–diagonal is shown in *frames 19* and *20*. The occluded right coronary artery was then treated with balloon pre-dilatation (*frame 22*). Subsequently, one single long Cypher stent was implanted (*frames 24* and *25*).

Message   This case illustrates the combination of debulking and stenting in a patient considered to be at very high risk of restenosis: a diabetic patient with long and diffusely diseased vessels. The association of IVUS evaluation, as said before, gives confidence that atherectomy can be performed at a distal vessel.

7. Restenosis after treatment of triple-vessel disease with multiple DES: do we need a new generation of DES?

Case # 10927/02

This is a typical example (**slides 1–9** (*frames 1–19*)) of triple-vessel disease in a patient with diabetes mellitus. There was a long area of diffused disease in the right coronary artery as demonstrated in *frames 1* and *2*. This vessel was treated with long Cypher-stent implantation with achievement of an optimal result (*frames 3* and *4*).

The next step was to address to the left coronary system. There was a significant disease at the origin of the diagonal branch, of the intermediate branch, and in the mid part of the circumflex. Unfortunately, the disease in the ostium of the intermediate branch posed a danger for the left main and for the bifurcation LAD–circumflex. The first step was to deploy a Cypher stent in the mid part of the circumflex as shown in *frame 6*. The results were reasonably satisfactory as shown in *frame 7*.

Attention was then turned to the LAD and diagonal, where two stents were implanted in a crushing fashion from the diagonal into the LAD and then with a Cypher-stent deployment in the LAD. The final result at this level is shown in *frame 10*. The next step was to address the bifurcation at the ostial LAD and ostial intermediate. This time, we elected to utilize the V-technique, which appears relatively simple and straightforward, particularly when there is no need to create a proximal carina which continues quite proximally to the original carina. This approach gave a very good result at the level of the intermediate branch and the LAD, while there was a residual stenosis at the level of the circumflex. The final step was to wire this vessel as shown in *frame 14* and place a short Cypher stent. The final result appeared very satisfactory, as shown in *frame 15*. It is important to mention that in this particular case we did not perform final kissing balloon inflation. *Frame 16* shows the final result at the level of the right coronary artery.

Unfortunately, the early follow-up, trigged by new symptoms, showed an unusually aggressive restenosis at the distal left main and at the ostium of the circumflex and intermediate branch. There was diffuse disease in the mid and distal part of the right coronary artery. Owing to the aggressive nature of this restenosis, this patient was then treated with coronary artery by-pass surgery.

Message   This case is interesting because it shows, in our view, some limitations of drug-eluting stents, particularly when used in certain patients with diabetes who may have an unusually aggressive reaction. It is difficult to believe that just a specific technical innovation in stent implantation technique would be sufficient to prevent this problem. The pattern of restenosis was diffuse and not just focal – a situation which is more likely to be technically related.

We will be waiting for the next generation of drug-eluting stents.

8. More puzzles after multivessel stenting with DES

Case # 10845/02

Case # 10845/02 is illustrated by slides 1–8 (*frames 1–21*). The patient presented with unprotected left main disease and multiple lesions at the level of the left system (*frames 1–3*) and at the level of the right coronary artery (*frame 4*). *Frame 3* shows the extent of the diffuse disease at the level of the small circumflex coronary artery.

Treatment started with the left anterior descending, which was treated with multiple Cypher stents and balloon dilatation of a diagonal branch (*frames 5–8*). The next vessel to be treated was the diffusely diseased circumflex, which was treated with two Cypher stents (*frames 9* and *10*) following vessel pre-dilatation. The last Cypher stent placed in the circumflex was crushed by a stent in the left anterior descending (*frames 11* and *12*) in order to treat the left main lesion. The final result is shown in *frames 13* and *14*.

The right coronary artery was then addressed with pre-dilatation and then cutting balloon angioplasty. It is conceivable that other factors, rather than technical reasons, were involved in the decision not to implant a Cypher stent at this level. The 6-months follow-up, shows a focal restenosis in the mid of the left main coronary artery, as demonstrated in *frames 18* and *19*.

Message   It is somewhat puzzling to see restenosis in a rather large vessel without any restenosis in more distal locations – sites that are theoretically more prone to this event – including the right coronary artery which was treated without stenting (as shown in *frame 21*). This case illustrates a current dilemma: why does restenosis occur in a patient at a certain level and not at other sites?

9. Fx Minirail for lesion preparation

Case # 11532/03

This case (slides 1–7 (*frames 1 17*)) illustrates a patient with a lesion involving the distal part of the left main trunk extending into the proximal and mid LAD. The lesion involved the proximal part of the bifurcation from which a large diagonal originates (*frame 2*).

Being a long lesion with diffused disease, we preferred to take a strategy to pre-dilate fully the lesion in order to allow a better stent expansion. In this particular case, we decided to use a balloon Fx Minirail (Guidant) (3.5 × 10 mm). This balloon is a slight modification of the cutting balloon, but with improved flexibility. It is important to note that we did not use an undersized balloon, but we used a 3.5-mm balloon in order to pre-dilate fully the lesion and break any fibrotic part or any calcium, which could endanger the homogeneous stent expansion. For this reason, a dissection is clearly present in *frame 5*. We do not fear the presence of a dissection if we know in advance that we are going to place a stent. As a matter of fact, the presence of the dissection is a guarantee that the lesion has been fully dilated. The distal part of the LAD was treated first with a 3.5 × 18-mm Cypher stent, while a wire was in the circumflex (*frame 6*). The results in the RAO projection are shown in *frame 7*.

The reason why the diagonal was not protected or treated is because the ostium of the diagonal had no disease; the disease was present mainly in the proximal part of the bifurcation (pseudo-bifurcation type lesion).

The next step was to treat the left main lesion as shown in *frame 8*. For this procedure, we selected the crush technique. As mentioned on a number of occasions, the advantage of this technique is its safety and the fact that the operator never loses access to either of the two branches. When dealing with an unprotected left main trunk, this last concept is of foremost importance. A 3.5-mm Cypher stent was advanced from the left main into the LAD following prior advancement of a 3.5 × 33-mm Cypher stent into the circumflex. In this case, we selected to crush the stent in the circumflex from the Cypher in the LAD. However, this rule is not fixed, and sometimes the operator can decide instead to do an inverted crush and to crush the LAD stent with the circumflex stent. What it is important and should never be forgotten is that the stent which is finally inflated most always be the most proximal stent, not the most distal one. The steps of the crush procedure are presented in *frames 8–10*.

Frame 8 verifies the position of the two stents as documented by a cine angiogram. *Frame 9* shows inflation of the stent in the circumflex clearly protruding into the left main for a few millimeters. *Frame 10* shows deployment of the stent in the LAD following removal of the balloon and the wire from the circumflex. Before inflating the stent into the LAD, we always take an angiogram to evaluate better the result in the circumflex. This step is important in order to be certain that no additional stent is needed in the distal circumflex.

Frames 11 and *12* show the results of the procedure in the left main trunk and in the proximal LAD. What is not shown in this case is the final kissing, which we always recommend even if the final result appears more than satisfactory.

Another possible way of treating this lesion could have been to utilize the V- or kissing-stent technique. When dealing with bifurcational lesions of the left main, particularly with a short left main or any left main length but without disease in the body, the V-technique is fast and easy. We still do not know the outcome of this technique in terms of angiographic restenosis. Preliminary reports indicate that it is safe.

The next step was to treat one discrete lesion in the mid part of the right coronary artery. The more proximal lesion demonstrated in *frame 13* was not considered to be significant. The fact that this lesion was focal and no calcium was seen on the angiogram prompted us to proceed with direct stenting (*frame 14*) utilizing a 3.5×20-mm Taxus stent. The final result is demonstrated in *frame 15*. More than the final result what is rewarding is the 6-month angiographic follow-up demonstrated in *frames 16* and *17* with excellent patency for the proximal LAD, distal left main and mid right coronary artery. The proximal lesion in the right coronary artery does not seem to have progressed.

Message This case illustrates the value of lesion pre-dilatation and appropriate preparation when dealing with a complex anatomy and with diffused disease and the utilization of a simple technique like direct stenting when the lesion is not complex to simplify the procedure.

10. Multiple bifurcations and diffuse disease

Case # 10663/03

This case (slides 1–8 (*frames 1–22*)) illustrates the treatment of multivessel coronary disease in a patient with a chronically occluded right coronary artery considered not suitable for PCI. *Frame 1* shows disease in the circumflex: a bifurcational lesion of the obtuse marginal branch (OM). *Frame 2* is interesting because it shows collateralization of the LAD through the conus branch visible just before the occlusion site of the right coronary artery. The strategy utilized in this case was first to dilate the circumflex. Being a complex multivessel disease, we performed pre-dilatation of the lesion as shown in *frames 3* and *4*, and the results following pre-dilatation are shown in *frame 5*.

The next step was to treat the bifurcation, which was stented utilizing the crush technique. Two Cypher stents, 3.0 and 2.5 mm, were inserted in the OM and in the circumflex, regarding the distal circumflex as the main branch. There was some debate as to whether to proceed and stent also the lesion in the distal circumflex toward the postero-lateral branches, but this decision was not taken and the lesion was not treated.

Frame 8 illustrates the important final step, which is now routine in the performance of the crush technique: final kissing inflation following rewiring of the side branch.

The next procedure was the treatment of the distal bifurcational lesion of the left main following wiring of the left anterior descending. It is not routine in our experience, but in this case with diffused disease and considerable plaque, we preferred to perform atherectomy of the ostium of the LAD and the distal left main in order to obtain a better stent expansion. The post-DCA result is shown in *frame 12*. It is evident that any stent which is expanded in this artery following plaque removal will perform better, particularly if the stent is a drug-eluting stent. The result, which appeared favorable at the ostium of the circumflex, prompted us to proceed with stenting only towards the LAD, as demonstrated in *frame 13*. The post-stent result shows only a minimal effect at the ostium of the circumflex, which was not considered satisfactory for such a patient.

We proceeded with the technique of reverse crush, which is basically a provisional crush technique. This technique was performed following pre-dilatation of the struts towards the circumflex. The next step is illustrated in *frame 15* where a Cypher stent was advanced towards the circumflex with partial protrusion in the left main. At the same time, another balloon was inserted into the proximal LAD distal left main. The stent was inflated and the balloon was then utilized to crush the protruding part of the stent. This step is not shown in the frames. What is important in this technique is that following stent deployment into the circumflex and before inflation of the balloon in the LAD, the operator must completely remove the balloon and the wire from the circumflex.

The next step was to rewire the circumflex and re-advance a balloon in the circumflex. As usual, the re-advancement of a balloon in the circumflex may require utilization of a very low-profile balloon such as a Maverick 1.5 mm (Boston Scientific), which is necessary to pre-dilate partially the struts and to allow the passage of an appropriately sized balloon in order to perform the final kissing inflation as demonstrated in *frame 16*. The final result of the procedure in the proximal LAD and distal left main is shown in *frame 17*.

The next step was to treat a mid lesion in the left anterior descending. This appears to be an unconventional approach, because usually we prefer to treat the distal lesion first and then the proximal lesion. However, as the patient had a significant left main disease and considering that the anatomy of the distal LAD and mid LAD was not complex, we elected to proceed in a different way. The treatment of the mid-LAD lesion is demonstrated in *frames 18* and *19*; initially, we placed an 18-mm-long Cypher stent and then an 8-mm-long Cypher stent to treat a more distal lesion.

The final result is shown in *frames 20* and *21*.

At the 22-month follow-up, this patient remained asymptomatic with a negative exercise test despite the total occlusion of the right coronary artery. The double antiplatelet therapy was totally stopped after 14 months of uninterrupted use.

Message This is a typical case of multivessel disease with bifurcations and diffuse disease in the main vessel. The use of the crush technique allows simultaneous treatment of the bifurcation and of all segments with diffuse disease, particularly if located proximally to the bifurcation.

11. Multiple chronic dissections

Case # 11729/03

This case (**slides 1–10** (*frames 1–24*) and **slides 11, 12**) illustrates treatment of an unusual pathology, which is multivessel disease in a young gentleman with stable angina and a history of systemic lupus erythematosus. The angiogram shows multiple dissections with partial healing at the level of the circumflex and occlusion of the LAD with a proximal appearance that is reasonably similar to the circumflex. The right coronary artery, which is not demonstrated in this angiogram, is patent with multiple dissections.

The first step was to cannulate this circumflex and advance a wire in this artery with multiple dissections. Usually, the approach we take in this situation is to break the dissection towards the large distal lumen. This risk is usually taken without much complication because, following balloon inflation, the dissection communicates again with the true lumen. The wire utilized for this procedure is a Whisper wire (Guidant), which is sometimes advanced in the dissection plain but is then re-entered distally. Following wiring of both branches, balloon dilatation is performed, initially with a small balloon and then more confidently with a larger balloon. *Frame 5* illustrates the result following balloon dilatation. It is evident that there is further dissection but the distal lumen is effectively perfused. This procedure always involves a risk of losing some side branch, but this is an inevitable consequence. The dilatation is then completed with placement of the Cypher stent in the obtuse marginal branch and then into the distal circumflex. The bifurcation is treated in the usual manner utilizing a crush technique, as demonstrated in *frame 11*, and final kissing, which is not shown in these slides. The final result is demonstrated in *frames 14* and *15*.

The only branch that has been lost in this recanalization procedure is a secondary obtuse marginal branch, which originated in the mid part of the large obtuse branch. It is interesting that in a later frame (*frame 16*), a branch comes back that was not demonstrated in *frame 14*.

The next step was the treatment of the left anterior descending. Following Whisper wiring, the dissection plain was treated with multiple cuts utilizing a Silverhawk atherectomy catheter (Foxhollow), as demonstrated in *frame 18*. This procedure always carries with it some risk, but if IVUS is performed prior to the atherectomy and demonstrates that the artery is of sufficient diameter, the procedure can be performed with safety. Following atherectomy, the angiogram shows a diffusely diseased LAD, relatively small in size without many branches and with reconstitution of the true lumen as supported by visualization of multiple side branches in the distal and mid LAD (*frame 19*).

The next step was to stent the left anterior descending with Cypher stents. Being a diffused-disease vessel with a relatively good size distal lumen, we elected to stent only the proximal part of the vessel, utilizing one 3.5 × 33-mm Cypher stent. Even if not widely used, this is an example of spot drug-eluting stenting, which sometimes can be utilized instead of paving the entire left anterior descending.

The final result is demonstrated in *frames 23* and *24*, which show good reconstitution of the circumflex with reappearance of the secondary obtuse marginal branch and a satisfactory size of the proximal LAD, with some residual lesion in the mid and distal LAD. This could be treated at the follow-up if the clinical situation suggested this approach. **Slides 11** and **12** demonstrate the histological appearance of the tissue retrieved from the LAD during atherectomy. Both fresh and old thrombi are apparent, laid at the site of the atherosclerotic plaque. An unusual appearance is the presence of abundant lymphocytes inside the thrombi, which confirm the inflammatory nature of this lesion – a finding that is not so common in many atherosclerotic lesions.

Message   Wiring of a vessel with chronic dissections may require building a new track among the various flaps, trying to re-enter as early as possible in the true lumen.

5

Special Subsets

Drug-eluting stents for in-stent restenosis

1. Restenosis following crush treated with another crush

Case # 11186/02

This case illustrates an example of diffuse and unexpected failure following implantation of drug-eluting stents (**slides 1–6** (*frames 1–15* and *run 1*)). The baseline frame (*frame 1*) illustrates the index procedure, while *frame 2* illustrates the result following extensive reconstruction of the bifurcation of the circumflex and obtuse marginal branch utilizing Cypher stents (Cordis) and the crush technique. The follow-up result at 10 months surprisingly shows a sustained patency on the bifurcation with some narrowing, but multiple restenosis involving the distal circumflex and the distal portion of the obtuse marginal branch with a total occlusion of the most distal Cypher stent (*frame 4*). The procedure was repeated utilizing aggressive pre-dilatation with short cutting balloons as illustrated in *frames 5* and *6*. Following this pre-dilatation, we re-established good forward flow as shown in *frame 7*. The in-stent restenosis was then treated with a Taxus stent (Boston Scientific) utilizing a unique approach of crush over previous crush. This is demonstrated in *frames 8* and *9*, with the result shown in *frame 10*. In this case, final kissing balloon was utilized. Owing to the presence of residual narrowing in the distal part of the obtuse marginal branch, a small Taxus stent had to be advanced through the bifurcation distally. This is effectively demonstrated in *run 1*.

Message   This example is particularly interesting because it shows that when the bifurcation is effectively dilated, especially with kissing, a stent can be negotiated through the struts and advanced distally – even through the Cypher stent deployed earlier in the distal obtuse marginal branch. The procedure then was completed with implantation of a stent in the more proximal circumflex, yielding a very satisfactory result as shown in *frames 14* and *15*.

2. Restenosis following V-stenting treated with another V-stenting

Case # 10745/02

This is a case (**slides 1–4** (*frames 1–8*)) of restenosis occurring following implantation of a Sirolimus-eluting stent treated with a paclitaxel-polymer-eluting stent.

The baseline lesion is illustrated in *frame 1* and involves a protected left main bifurcational lesion. The index procedure was performed utilizing a V-technique owing to the fact that the left main coronary artery appeared short. There was implantation of a long stent towards the large circumflex and a short stent towards the stump of the left anterior descending. The final result following implantation of three Cypher stents is shown in *frame 4*. The follow-up at 10 months, when the patient returned because of symptoms, shows a severe focal restenosis at the ostium of the left anterior descending and two focal restenosis inside the Cypher stents in the circumflex, proximal, and mid-parts. The approach was to implant two Taxus stents utilizing a V-technique at the level of the bifurcation of the left main. Simple balloon angioplasty was performed in the more distal lesion of the circumflex.

At the 7-month follow-up, the patient was asymptomatic.

Message   The V-technique remains one of the fastest approaches to distal left main bifurcational disease.

3. Ostial diagonal lesions: always a difficult problem

Case # 10815/02

This is a case of ostial restenosis at the ostium of a diagonal branch treated with a Cypher stent (**slides 1–8** (*frames 1–16*)). As previously illustrated, the index lesion was treated with atherectomy and stenting (*frames 1* and *2* baseline). *Frames 3* and *4* are following the index procedure. At that time, a stent was placed at the ostium of a diagonal branch utilizing a T-technique. It is worth mentioning that at the time of the index procedure, the left anterior descending was treated with atherectomy and with bare-metal stent implantation. The follow-up angiogram at 8 months showed excellent maintained results at the level of the bare-metal stent in the left anterior descending and focal restenosis at the ostium of the diagonal branch. This restenosis was confirmed by IVUS, which showed that the stent appeared well deployed, but the lumen encroached by severe hyperplasia. An examination of *frame 7*, which is the IVUS at the time of the ostial restenosis at the diagonal branch, shows marked positive remodeling at the ostium of the diagonal branch with a vessel which is almost 3.75 mm in diameter. This occurrence is fairly rare.

The operator originally under-dilated the ostium of the diagonal branch. When this large amount of remodeling is present, the correct approach is not always clear, and dilatation to the appropriate size may become dangerous with the risk of vessel rupture. It is possible that these cases may need debulking extended at the ostium of the diagonal prior to stenting. Again, it is interesting that this approach was undertaken when the index lesion was treated, and perhaps the debulking was insufficient for the amount of plaque originally present. Whatever the explanation, we are facing a persistent limitation in some cases of stenting bifurcational lesions. The second procedure was performed with implantation of a 3-mm Taxus stent from the

LAD towards the diagonal. The stent was then crossed with a wire and dilated with a Maverick 3.5-mm balloon (*frame 10*). A kissing inflation was then performed as in the standard culottes technique. Owing to the presence of a distal dissection, two Taxus stents had to be implanted in the mid and distal left anterior descending. The IVUS evaluation performed at the ostium of the diagonal branch then revealed an optimal result with a stent expanded to a cross-sectional area of 7.3 mm^2.

Message It is impossible, but certainly intriguing, to conceive that if this excellent result were achieved at the time of original procedure, the risk of restenosis at the ostium of the diagonal branch would have been lower. It is important to point out that any approach to over-dilate ostial lesions in the diagonal branch always needs to be undertaken with IVUS evaluation, because this type of lesion can lead to vessel rupture if too aggressively treated.

4. Double dosing for a high-risk lesion

Case # 11055/02

This case (slides 1–3 (*frames 1–5*)) illustrates treatment of a rare but complex situation: a target-vessel failure following multiple procedures in a young patient with a history of three prior angioplasties, including brachytherapy in the distal left main and proximal left anterior descending. *Frame 1* illustrates a severe stenosis in the body of the left main. In order to achieve optimal dosing, the decision was taken to implant electively two Cypher stents (3×18 mm and 3×8 mm) at the level of the left main. An alternative solution could have been to utilize the seven-cell 3.5-mm Cypher stent instead of the two stents with six cells. At that time, the seven-cell stent was not yet available. The immediate result is excellent, as shown in *frame 4*.

More rewarding is the follow-up result, which shows an asymptomatic patient and the sustained patency of the index lesion.

Message This unusual approach, called the sandwich technique, has been utilized in a few patients with excellent follow-up results. The indication for this approach is multiple failures in high-risk lesions in which a higher density of strut coverage and dosage of the drug may be necessary. The fact that no case sustained a complication, including early or late thrombosis, supports the relatively large therapeutic windows that the Cypher stent has regarding the dosing of rapamycin.

5. Sirolimus-eluting stent for diffuse in-stent restenosis

Case # 29429HSR

This case (slide 1 (*frames 1–3*)) illustrates the new usage of drug-eluting stents, in the treatment of diffused in-stent restenosis. As shown in *frame 1*, there is a diffuse in-stent restenosis in the mid of the left anterior descending. In the past, this type of lesion was treated with cutting balloon and brachytherapy. This specific case has been treated with a simplified approach involving a long Cypher stent (33×3 mm) implantation in the mid of the LAD. The final result is shown in *frame 2*, and the follow-up result, with almost no late loss and preservation of the ostium of the diagonal, is presented in *frame 3*. This type of result gives encouragement to our approach to treat in-stent restenosis with a simplified format such as drug-eluting stent implantation, even for the diffuse type of in-stent restenosis.

Message   If this approach to the treatment of diffuse in-stent restenosis proves effective, there will be no reason to have any brachytherapy.

6. Repeat restenosis occurring at the same site

Case # 23753HSR

This case (**slides 1–6** (*frames 1–17*)) is unusual and interesting because it demonstrates repeat restenosis occurring following implantation of drug-eluting stents. This repeat restenosis occurred almost always at the same site, stressing most probably a mechanical and local issue. This patient had previously undergone extensive reconstruction of the left anterior descending, and we see a follow-up angiogram in *frame 1* demonstrating a focal restenosis in the mid and left anterior descending. At that time, a Cypher stent (18×3 mm) was implanted (*frames 2* and *3*) with a good final result (*frame 4*). The follow-up angiogram 6 months later showed persistence of good patency. The 12-month angiographic follow-up, owing to new symptoms, showed a lumen loss at that level, demonstrating a possibly significant stenosis. At that time, the patient was treated mainly because of his symptoms, even if, angiographically, the stenosis in *frames 6* and *7* appeared borderline. A Taxus stent (3×28 mm) was implanted, achieving an optimal result as shown in *frame 9*. Because of the occurrence of new symptoms, a 5-month angiographic follow-up was carried out, again demonstrating lumen loss at the same site (note the relation to the septal branch inside the Taxus stent) (*frames 11* and *12*).

At that time, a new angioplasty was performed without implanting any new stent and achieving an optimal result in December 2003 with a sustained patency in a mid-term follow-up angiography in March 2004. The IVUS image, which is shown in *frame 16*, shows fibrosis and calcification at the site of the repeated restenosis, stressing the importance of stent under-expansion at this level. In addition, *frame 16* shows that it may not be the calcium *per se*, but the calcium as a possible cause of stent under-expansion. It is intriguing that all the restenotic events occurred at the same site in the mid and left anterior descending.

7. Cypher for subacute Taxus stent thrombosis

Case # 11789/03

This case is illustrated by slides 1–5 (*frames 1–16*). The initial target lesion was located in the obtuse marginal branch as shown in *frame 1* and represented a restenosis inside the bare-metal stent. A Taxus stent (3 × 18 mm) was positioned, with an acceptable final result shown in *frame 3*. (Notice that there is a residual lesion in the very distal segment of the obtuse marginal branch.) Perhaps owing to the distal residual lesion or insufficient distal run-off, 1 month later the patient presented with new angina, without acute events, and the angiogram demonstrated occlusion of the stent as shown in *frame 4*. This is not a clinically evident thrombosis, but it is very suggestive. The vessel was reopened and pre-dilated as shown in *frame 6*. Intravascular ultrasound demonstrated a gross mismatch between the assumed vessel size in the initial procedure, where we assumed that the vessel was 3 mm in diameter, while the real vessel size was more than 4 mm in the proximal part and 3.8 mm in the mid-part. Note that there is distal diffuse disease in the obtuse marginal branch. This evaluation prompted the use of much larger and longer stents, and the final result demonstrated in *frame 13* was optimal. The intravascular ultrasound demonstrated a very large cross-sectional area and a reasonably symmetric apposition of the stent struts. At the 6 months clinical follow-up, the patient was asymptomatic.

Treatment of saphenous vein grafts and left internal mammary artery

1. Use of distal protection for saphenous vein graft treatment

Case # 11451/03

This case (slides 1–3 (*frames 1–4* and *runs 1, 2*)) illustrates a very proximal stenosis in a saphenous vein graft, which appeared relatively healthy for the other part of the graft. It is fairly rare to see degeneration at the ostium of a saphenous vein graft. As a matter of fact, many interventionists do not advocate use of protection devices for ostial saphenous vein-graft lesions. This lesion was not a pure ostial lesion, but a very proximal lesion, and the presence of a round feeling defect suggestive of thrombus is clear from *frame 1*. This particular circumstance prompted us to use a distal protection device. The very small residual lumen available for passage prompted us to choose the GuardWire (Medtronic) (*frame 2*). This device is still the protection device with the smallest profile, and was therefore less likely to dislodge the clot. The procedure was then followed by direct implantation of a 3.5×28-mm Taxus stent (Boston Scientific). Following aspiration and deflation of the guide-wire, the final result is shown in *run 2*, with excellent distal TIMI flow as well as a good result at the site of the stenosis as seen in *frame 4*.

Message   The message for this case is that with almost all, if not all, types of saphenous vein-graft lesions, we nowadays need a form of distal protection during interventions.

2. Treatment of an occluded saphenous vein graft: stents covered with bovine pericardium plus DES

Case # 11674/03

This is an example (slides 1–9 (*frames 1–13* and *runs 1–8*)) of a total occluded saphenous vein graft, which again illustrates the value of combining distal protection with anti-restenotic technology. The graft was on the right coronary artery and appeared occluded. Following passage of a wire, a PercuSurge protection device (Medtronic) was positioned in the distal part of the graft. Sometimes a wise maneuver is to probe the distal circulation with a multifunctional probing catheter to inject and evaluate the size of the distal bed. This procedure is usually helpful before embarking on a complex reopening of a saphenous vein graft, which may supply a very small and diffusely diseased distal bed. *Frames 1* and *2* illustrate the PercuSurge and balloon angioplasty with protection by the inflated PercuSurge balloon. Note the shape of the PercuSurge balloon, which is quadrangular, attesting the optimal inflation of this balloon with good sealing.

Following initial aspiration of the thrombotic material and various inflations, the PercuSurge balloon was deflated and a check was performed. This angiogram requires deflation of the PercuSurge balloon in order to evaluate the next steps to be carried out. The arrow in *frame 1* points towards a residual lesion in the distal body of the graft, while the two arrows (*frame 3*) show residual lesions in the proximal part of the graft. The PercuSurge balloon is inflated again, and two stents covered with bovine pericardium are deployed in the proximal and mid part of the graft. The aspiration is performed and the PercuSurge balloon is deflated to evaluate again (*run 3*). The proximal and distal segments of the stents are then sealed by implanting a Cypher stent (Cordis) (3.5×27 mm) in order to protect against edge restenosis. The very distal lesion is treated with another 3.5-mm stent covered with bovine pericardium. It is interesting to take into account how this very slippery stent negotiates inside the proximal deployed stents despite its rather large profile. *Run 4* shows the result after deployment of the more distal pericardium stent. A subsequent Cypher stent (3.5×23 mm) is deployed in the more distal part. The only segment that is left uncovered is a segment between the distal bovine-pericardium-covered stent and the intermediate Cypher stent. The procedure is finally completed by positioning a 4-mm bovine-pericardium-covered stent at the ostium of the saphenous vein graft.

The final result is shown in *run 6*, which demonstrates a total reconstruction of the graft. It is more interesting to see the angiographic follow-up at 5 months (*runs 7* and *frame 10*) which show a gap restenosis right distally to a Cypher stent. It is remarkable how this complete graft reconstruction has been able to maintain optimal patency with a very minimal and focal restenosis in a short segment. This focal restenosis was treated with implantation of a 3.5×18-mm Cypher stent. The final result is demonstrated in *run 8*.

Message   It is remarkable to see both the immediate result and the follow-up result, which mean that we no longer need to resist the temptation to reopen occluded saphenous vein grafts when the distal bed is functionally and anatomically adequate.

3. Treatment of an occluded saphenous vein graft

Case # 11631/03

This is an example of contemporary treatment of an occluded saphenous vein graft (slides 1–8 (*frames 1–10* and *runs 1–4*)). In the past, there was a reluctance to reopen these vessels for two reasons: first, complications related to the procedures, and second, poor probabilities of maintaining long-term patency.

At the present time, some of these concerns seem to have declined. Following crossing of the occlusion with a wire, we examined the situation. The graft appeared with diffuse disease or loaded with thrombus. At this point, an occlusive device such as a guide-wire was put into the distal position, angioplasty was performed proximally and an X-Sizer (EndiCOR Medical) was advanced into the graft in order to remove material of thrombus (*frame 3*).

Run 3 and *frame 4* show the result following the X-Sizer procedure. At this point, in order to maintain the better visualization necessary for accurate stent positioning, the protection device was switched with the Epi Filter wire (Boston Scientific). Under Epi Filter wire protection, three Taxus stents were positioned (*frames 5–7*). Still with a filter in place, it is possible to perform an injection which shows a residual filling defect in the distal part of the right coronary artery and a very proximal defect in the initial portion of the saphenous vein graft (*frame 8*). A 32-mm Taxus stent is finally implanted at the proximal portion, and a 32×3-mm stent is implanted in the most distal position. The final result is shown in *run 4*, which demonstrates not only an optimal lumen throughout the saphenous vein graft but also a surprising TIMI 3 flow at the level of the distal bed.

4. Sandwich technique for ostial saphenous vein graft

Case # 10901/02

This is an unusual case of resilient ostial restenosis in a saphenous vein graft (**slides 1–6** (*frames 1–15*)). The importance of the saphenous vein graft (SVG) will be understood when examining the large distribution territory of this conduit.

The history of this lesion starts in the year 2000 with the implantation of a Bestent (Medtronic) at the ostium. Following restenosis, a PTFE-covered stent was then implanted in an attempt to seal any hyperplasia. Unfortunately, a new restenosis occurred in 2001. At that time, a simple bare-metal stent was implanted. Following a new restenosis, the lesion was treated with an aggressive implantation of two Cypher stents according to the sandwich technique. This is demonstrated in *frames 2–4* which show an excellent final result. Unfortunately, despite this aggressive approach, a new restenosis occurred as shown in *frames 7* and *8*. The procedure was then undertaken with a pre-dilatation with a cutting balloon and a 'combined' chemotherapy utilizing a Taxus and a Cypher stent and implanted according to a sandwich technique again (*frame 11*). The final result is shown in *frame 13* following implantation of an additional Cypher stent more distally to treat a residual lesion. This patient was asymptomatic at the 7-month clinical follow-up, and hopefully we will obtain angiographic follow-up.

Message   Again this case shows that when clinically indicated, persistence can be of help, and a combination of multiple drug-eluting stents is certainly an area to be explored in selected cases in which surgical revascularization does not appear a good option.

5. Flow deterioration in a saphenous vein graft

Case # 34552HSR

This case exemplifies various issues (**slides 1–5** (*frames 1–5 and runs 1–5*)). One is the occurrence of no-reflow which has been misdiagnosed as a proximal obstruction. This fact triggered treatment of the proximal segment of the saphenous vein graft rather than treating the no-reflow. The baseline *frame 1* and *run 1* show a lesion in the mid part of the saphenous vein graft to the right coronary artery, with excellent TIMI 3 flow. Following direct stent implantation, there was a reduction of the flow to TIMI 2 as demonstrated in *run 2*. The operator believed that the reduction in distal flow was the result of the presence of proximal disease and proceeded with implantation of another stent more proximally, as demonstrated in *frame 3*. The subsequent injection (*frame 4*) shows what was clearly expected, which is a further reduction of flow, now without opacification of the distal bed. The diffuse disease present proximally was again interpreted as a possible cause of this flow reduction, and another stent was implanted in the more proximal part. At this point, there was a further more dramatic reduction of distal flow (*run 4*). Finally, an infusion catheter, such as the multifunctional probing catheter, was selectively advanced in the graft (*frame 5*) and nitroprusside 200 μg was selectively injected through the multifunctional probing catheter. There was an impressively prompt restoration of TIMI 3 flow as seen in *run 5*. Again, this case illustrates the importance to recognize a problem quickly and to treat it appropriately.

Message   A flow deterioration during treatment of a saphenous vein graft is due to distal embolization until proven otherwise.

6. A retrograde rescue of a mammary artery

Case # 10696/02

This case, which could be called rescuing the mammary by passing from the left anterior descending, is illustrated by **slides 1–9** (*frames 1–10 and runs 1–9*). *Run 1* shows a not well-functioning mammary artery anastomosed to the mid left anterior descending. *Frame 1* shows a diffusely diseased LAD, which appears occluded in the distal part at the site of insertion of the mammary artery.

The first step was to dilate the native LAD at the level of the lesion in the mid portion and improve the situation at the bifurcation of the diagonal branch. A Cypher 2.5-mm stent was implanted in the mid part in order to facilitate the distal visualization, despite the fact that the distal vessel cannot be seen, and the site of the occlusion is demonstrated by the arrow in *frame 5*. At this point, the operator was lucky to advance a wire from the LAD into the mammary artery as shown in *frame 6*, and a dilatation was performed towards the mammary artery in order to improve the flow in this vessel. The results after the dilatation are shown in *run 4*, which demonstrates visualization of the distal LAD. Clearly, there was some compromise at the site of the anastomosis towards the distal LAD.

Following additional balloon inflations, disease in the distal LAD right after the anastomosis appeared more clearly (*frame 8*). At this point, advancement of the wire from the mammary into the distal LAD was performed, and an 18×2.5-mm Cypher stent was positioned in the distal left anterior descending. The angiogram demonstrated in *run 6* shows the mammary, and *run 7* shows patency from the native left anterior descending. The 10-month follow-up, even if not performed with a selective injection in the LIMA graft, showed sustained patency of the LIMA with visualization of the distal LAD and maintained patency of the native LAD. There was no visualization of the distal LAD, most probably due to competitive flow at this level. There is a lesion in the proximal part of the LAD, which was never treated at the index procedure and was not treated during this follow-up procedure due to the excellent clinical conditions of the patient.

Message   The main message of this case is that a mammary can sometimes be rescued by passing from the native vessels.

7. Understanding the anatomy of a saphenous vein graft while reopening

Case # 11903/04

This case illustrates problem solving in a difficult anatomy of the saphenous vein graft (**slides 1–7** (*frames 1–16 and runs 1–5*)). *Run 1* shows a saphenous vein graft to a diagonal branch, while *frame 1* shows the native anatomy with occlusion of the circumflex and bridging collateral; the LAD is occluded after a first septal branch.

The operator advanced a wire from the LAD and back into a saphenous vein graft as shown in *frame 2*. As it will appear later in *run 2*, this saphenous vein graft is connected to the saphenous vein graft to the diagonal branch, and it is basically a portion of a jump graft from the diagonal into the left anterior descending. The procedure continued with dilatation of the proximal LAD as shown in *frames 3–5*. The result after balloon dilatation is presented in *frame 6*. Higher-pressure dilatation was performed with the Powersail balloon (Guidant) as demonstrated in *frames 7* and *8*, and again the lesion preparation was completed as shown in *run 3*. The proximal LAD was then treated with implantation of three Taxus stents, and the result is demonstrated in *run 4*. From this injection, the jump part of the graft can be faintly visualized, showing that the graft goes from the LAD to the diagonal branch. *Frames 12* and *13* show completion of dilation of the proximal LAD and maintained patency of the septal branch. A final short stent was implanted at the ostium of a septal branch in order to maintain patency on this important vessel, as shown in *frames 14* and *16* with post-dilatation of this stent. The result is shown in *run 5* with a wire again positioned in the graft of the diagonal branch.

Message   The main message of this case is the usage of guide-wires to delineate anatomy in complex situations.

6
Special Procedures

Atherectomy and rotablation

1. Debulking with atherectomy before DES implantation: 'la crème de la crème'

Case # 11817/03

This case (**slides 1–8** (*frames 1–23*)) illustrates a lesion involving the proximal LAD and extending in the mid part of the vessel. The distal left main is free from disease, and the circumflex has a borderline lesion in the distal part (*frame 1*). *Frame 2* shows the lesion extending towards the proximal and mid LAD. The baseline IVUS assessment shows soft plaque in the proximal part of the lesion and fibro-calcific plaque in the most distal segment (illustrated in *frames 3–5*). The initial approach was to debulk partially this lesion with significant amount of plaque in order to allow optimal stent expansion. This procedure was also done to minimize possible plaque shift towards the circumflex. The device utilized was a large Silverhawk device (Foxhollow), compatible with the 8-Fr guide-catheter (*frame 8*). The result after atherectomy treatment shows a fair result in the proximal part with persistent stenosis in the distal part of the lesion. This stenosis corresponds to the area with fibro-calcific deposits at the IVUS evaluation. For this reason, cutting balloon dilatation was performed (*frame 11*), and then the atherectomy device could be advanced at that level. The final result was significantly better than before cutting balloon dilatation, and several atherectomy specimens were retrieved (*frame 14*).

The next step was to implant two long Taxus stents, 3.5 mm in diameter. It is interesting to note in *frames 18–20* that an optimal symmetry was achieved with excellent stent expansion, and all the branches maintained patency (*frame 21*). The ostium of the circumflex is not at all compromised (*frame 22*), and final lumen is excellent also in the cranial view (*frame 23*).

Message   Even if atherectomy should not be seen as an essential procedure when we treat an ostial LAD lesion, particularly when the plaque burden is very large, our threshold to use an associated technology is relatively low, and we still believe that the long-term results are likely to be superior if plaque removal and optimal stent extension is achieved.

2. LAD ostial lesion and plaque shift towards the circumflex

Case # 11091/02

This case is an example of an in-stent restenosis of an ostial LAD lesion (slides 1–6 (*frames 1–13*)). As shown in *frames 1* and *2*, this case highlights a typical problem that we face in the treatment of these lesions: plaque shift towards the circumflex.

The operator attempted to prevent this issue by performing atherectomy on the left anterior descending utilizing the Silverhawk device as demonstrated in *frames 3* and *4*. Following atherectomy, a gentle balloon dilatation was performed, and a Cypher stent was implanted at the ostium of the left anterior descending. The final result after Cypher implantation is shown in *frame 7*. Despite atherectomy, there was a plaque shift with narrowing at the ostium of the circumflex. The next step was to perform kissing balloon dilatation as demonstrated in *frame 8*; the result following the procedure is shown in *frame 9*. There is improvement at the level of the circumflex, but still some residual lesion. This residual lesion prompted the operator to implant a short stent at the ostium of the circumflex with a T-technique. The final result is shown in *frame 11*. This case illustrates the problem of plaque shift at the ostium of the circumflex when treating a proximal LAD lesion. Interestingly, this problem occurred despite atherectomy performed on the LAD; possibly the fact that the original lesion was an in-stent restenosis negated the advantage of atherectomy. The follow-up result demonstrated sustained patency with an absence of restenosis at the bifurcation level.

Message   The main message is that these ostial lesions are, on the whole, unpredictable. In some circumstances, plaque shift does not occur despite lack of debulking; at other times, plaque shift occurs despite debulking. The plaque shift can at times be corrected by performing simple balloon inflation, while in other circumstances a stent implantation becomes necessary. Unfortunately, no study is available addressing the advantage of lesion debulking in the prevention of plaque shift.

3. A severely calcified large vessel where rotablation is combined with cutting balloon

Case # 11628/03

This case (slides 1–5 (*frames 1–12*)) illustrates the combination of a long lesion involving a segment of the proximal and mid LAD with calcification and a severe tandem lesion. *Frames 1* and *2* demonstrate the index lesion. Owing to extensive calcification, the lesion was prepared with rotational atherectomy and then use of the cutting balloon to perform the most appropriate dilatation in these large vessels. The procedure was completed with the implantation of one long Taxus stent

(3.5×32 mm; *frame 8*). The final result is demonstrated in *frames 9* and *10*, with excellent final LAD. The follow-up at 8.5 months shows maintenance of full patency of the treated vessel.

Message A single case cannot be used to prove a hypothesis, but it is reasonably suggestive that in this case of extensive calcifications, long lesion and diffuse disease, the follow-up result was well maintained without any evidence even of focal renarrowing. It is conceivable that appropriate lesion preparation may have contributed to better stent expansion and more homogeneous drug delivery.

4. Rotablation and crushing with a 6-Fr guiding catheter (step-crush technique)

Case # 11718/03

As illustrated by slides 1–6 (*frames 1–15*) and slides 7–12, this is a bifurcational lesion of a left anterior descending with an in-stent restenosis of moderate severity in the mid LAD plus a severe narrowing of the diagonal branch. There is also disease of the circumflex as demonstrated in *frames 1* and *2*. The operator decided first to treat the most severe vessel, which is a diagonal, dilated first with a balloon. Owing to incomplete expansion of the balloon as demonstrated in *frame 4*, rotational atherectomy was then performed with subsequent complete expansion of the balloon as demonstrated in *frame 6*. The next step was to implant a stent in the diagonal branch with the idea not to stent the left anterior descending. The stent was made to protrude in the LAD, and the protruding part was crushed with a 2.75-mm Maverick balloon.

As will be seen later, the LAD was then stented and this procedure became a classic crushing technique, but now performed in a step fashion with the side branch stented first and the main branch stented second. Incidentally, this approach is sometimes utilized to perform the crushing technique when the operator has the availability of a 6-Fr guiding catheter only. As a matter of fact, this specific case was carried out from the radial artery, and a 6-Fr guiding catheter was utilized. Following implantation of the stent in the side branch, there was a crushing of the protruding part as shown in *frame 9* with the result shown in *frame 10*. A Taxus stent was then implanted in the LAD with another stent implanted more proximally. The final result is demonstrated in *frames 14* and *15*. This particular case was performed without final kissing.

Message The main message of this case is the illustration of what we call 'step crushing', which is a classic crushing technique performed utilizing a 6-Fr guiding catheter and stenting the diagonal first. Everything else is fairly similar, with stenting of the LAD performed after stenting the diagonal branch. At the present time, this procedure would be completed with final kissing on both branches.

5. Double-vessel atherectomy for bifurcational lesion

Case # 10815/02

This case (slides 1–6 (*frames 1–11*)) illustrates a complex bifurcation involving a diffusely diseased left anterior descending and a diagonal branch. The procedure was initiated by performing Silverhawk atherectomy on both vessels, diagonal and LAD. When this procedure is performed, the guide-wire needs to be removed from one of the two branches, and in this case there was a temporary occlusion of the diagonal branch as shown in *frame 6*. The diagonal was then reopened and atherectomy was performed in this vessel. The procedure was completed by implanting a long stent (Cypher 2.5×33 mm) at the diagonal branch, while a large-diameter bare-metal stent was implanted on the LAD. The decision to use a bare-metal stent was motivated by the fact that no large-diameter drug-eluting stent was available at that time. The result following the implantation of two stents is illustrated in *frames 7* and *8*; there is a clear residual stenosis at the ostium of the diagonal branch due to its incomplete coverage. The operator attempted to correct this problem by performing a kissing dilatation as shown in *frame 9*. The final result appeared very satisfactory. Unfortunately, this patient developed restenosis, which involved the ostium of the diagonal branch. The LAD maintained good patency. This residual lesion was then treated with drug-eluting stent implantation.

Message   Debulking appears to be an important procedure, particularly in diffusely diseased vessels. The sustained good result on the LAD substantiates the above statement. Unfortunately, the side branches are frequently not completely handled, and at times a focal stenosis can occur at the ostium of the side branch. Our opinion is that at the level of the side branch, the angulation defeats the possibility of performing effective debulking. Despite this event, we should not consider this focal stenosis a major failure because they are usually quite easy to re-treat.

6. Buddy-wire to enhance stent delivery

Case # 11899/04

This case (slides 1–9 (*frames 1–25*)) illustrates a severe triple-vessel disease characterized by unprotected left main with distal stenosis, multiple stenoses in the proximal and mid LAD, and total occlusion of the right coronary artery. *Frames 1* and *2* show the baseline coronary anatomy. This patient had a history of myasthenia gravis, and this fact was the main reason why he was not treated with a surgical revascularization. The LAD lesion was first approached with rotational atherectomy for two reasons. Firstly, the extensive calcifications may prevent effective dilatation, and secondly, the tortuosity of the LAD with calcification and the need to implant long stents necessitate optimal lesion preparation.

An associated clinical factor was the presence of hematoma during right femoral artery puncture. This complication did not allow the prophylactic insertion of an intra-aortic balloon pump. *Frame 3* shows the anatomy in the RAO projection at the time of rotablation of the LAD, and *frame 5* shows the result after rotablation with incomplete filling of the distal left anterior descending, suggesting slow flow. The patient was treated with balloon angioplasty in order to improve immediately flow in the distal LAD. This approach is very important, and it was almost routine at the time of use of the rotablator, when extensive and quick low-pressure balloon infla-tions appeared the best way to re-establish good flow in the distal vessel. *Frame 9* shows improved filling of the left anterior descending following balloon angioplasty. To facilitate stent advancement, the lesion was then prepared with Fx Minirail (Guidant; 3.0 mm) and high-pressure PowerSail balloon (Guidant) inflation. Note in *frames 10* and *11* the presence of an additional wire (buddy-wire) to support better the guiding catheter and the delivery balloon for stent placement. Stents were placed in the distal LAD and mid LAD with some difficulties, but finally with good coverage of the lesion (a 3-mm stent distally and a 3.5-mm stent proximally). The diagonal maintained patency, and there was no need to perform any procedure on this vessel. The proximal stent was deployed to cover the left main, and a provisional approach towards the circumflex was chosen (*frames 15–17*).

The next step was to improve the ostium of the circumflex with a kissing balloon inflation in order to avoid stenting of this vessel. The results in the RAO projection are shown in *frame 19*. The results after kissing showed some residual stenosis at the ostium of the circumflex (*frame 20*), a result not considered adequate. For this reason, the operator decided to proceed with stent implantation. Stents were implanted according to the reverse crushing technique because a stent was already in place in the left main and LAD. A balloon was used to crush the protruding part of a Taxus stent positioned in the circumflex. The steps of crushing, including recrossing, are shown in the various frames until *frame 23*. The final result is presented in *frames 24* and *25*.

Message   Lesion preparation is of the utmost importance in calcified tortuous lesions. The difficulties encountered in advancing the stents in the LAD despite prior rotablation, high-pressure balloon inflation including Fx Minirail usage and buddy-wire extra support show how complex stent delivery can be in some multivessel disease. The presence of a normal left ventricular function at baseline permitted performance of this procedure without elective intra-aortic balloon counterpulsation, which we strongly recommend despite the good outcome of this case.

IVUS guidance

1. IVUS guidance to increase final lumen cross-sectional area: a worthwhile effort?

Case # 11587/03

This is an example of IVUS usage in deployment of a drug-eluting stent (slides 1–17 (*frames 1–48*)). We are still unclear as to the advantage of optimizing stent expansion, but we would like to illustrate this case just to make the point that, with IVUS guidance, the lumen cross-sectional area is certainly larger, and the contact of the stent struts to the media is better, with a shorter distance from the struts to the media.

Frames 1 and *2* illustrate a lesion in the proximal circumflex in a somewhat large vessel by angiography, most probably 3.5 mm. The IVUS examination presented in *frames 4–6* shows that the vessel diameter is more than 4 mm in all the three frames. In view of these measurements, we used a 3.5×18-mm Cypher stent (Cordis) (if available, we would most probably have used a 4.0-mm Cypher). The results after direct stenting are illustrated in *frame 8*. The IVUS evaluation following stent expansion, which is shown in *frames 10–12*, demonstrates that in some sections, such as *frames 10* and *11*, the stent is still slightly under-expanded, with a large distance from the struts to the internal elastic lamina. For this reason, we post-dilated the stent with a 4-mm balloon as shown in *frames 13* and *14*. The IVUS evaluation following post-dilatation is shown in *frames 16–18*, and in *frames 19–21* we see the improvement from a cross-sectional area of $7 \, mm^2$ to $8.2 \, mm^2$ following post-dilatation with a 4-mm balloon. Again, we are uncertain of the impact of this improvement, but it is clear that with IVUS guidance we almost always obtain a larger final lumen.

The same patient underwent a procedure on a diagonal branch, as shown in *frames 24* and *25*, with a stenosis in the mid part of a small but long diagonal branch. The IVUS evaluation (*frames 27–29*) shows that at the site of the lesion there is a slight negative remodeling, with a vessel diameter of $<2.5 \, mm$ in one section. The proximal and distal segments are larger. We pre-dilated the lesion with a 2-mm diameter cutting balloon (as shown in *frame 31*) and then implanted a 23-mm Cypher stent with a diameter of 2.25 mm. The IVUS evaluation is presented in *frames 35–37*, while in the mid segment of lesion there is still a very small lumen cross-sectional area of $2.0 \, mm^2$. For this reason, we post-dilated this segment with a PowerSail balloon (Guidant; 2.5 mm in diameter) and re-evaluated with IVUS (*frame 42*), which now shows an increased cross-sectional area of $2.6 \, mm^2$. *Frames 44–46* show the improvement in cross-sectional area from baseline to 2.6 mm² following the PowerSail post-dilatation. Again, we do not know the impact of this change, but certainly in selected lesions this optimization may have a role. Until a prospective study is undertaken, we will not be able to answer this important question.

Message   IVUS evaluation almost always leads to a larger final cross-sectional area. We are uncertain as to the value of this extra gain when drug-eluting stents are implanted.

2. Many restenoses which occur at the site of a bifurcation are due to stent underexpansion and possibly stent recoil

Case # 11540/03

This case is illustrated by slides 1–5 (*frames 1–10*). The baseline projections (*frames 1 and 2*) show restenosis at the ostium of the left anterior descending; the circumflex originates with an acute angle. This situation makes this vessel very likely to be jeopardized following a stenting of the LAD. The operator first stented the LAD but then, owing to plaque shift towards the circumflex, he had to place a stent at the ostium of this vessel (as demonstrated in *frames 3* and *4*). The stent in the LAD was deployed first and then, following dilatation of the struts, a second short stent was advanced into the circumflex. The IVUS evaluation following kissing balloon inflation with a 3-mm balloon in the circumflex is demonstrated in *frame 5*, which shows a cross-sectional area at the ostium of the circumflex of 4.8 mm². This is clearly a small lumen, particularly when compared with the distal part of the stent (as shown in *frame 6*), where there is a cross-sectional area of 8.5 mm². This finding prompted usage of a larger balloon, and a kissing inflation was performed at high pressure with a 3.5-mm balloon. The angiographic results are better (as shown in *frame 8*) and the cross-sectional area at the ostium of the circumflex increased to 6.7 mm² (as demonstrated in *frame 9*).

Message   In these ostial lesions that are prone to recurrence even following drug-eluting stent implantation, we believe that this optimization is important.

3. Ostial left main and ostial LAD: value of IVUS and angiography

Case # 11948/04

This is a case (slides 1–5 (*frames 1–11*)) where there are two lesions: one lesion in the ostium of the left main and another possible lesion in the proximal left anterior descending. The ostial left main is easier to evaluate because of significant pressure damping upon insertion of the guiding catheter. *Frames 1* and *2* illustrate the baseline lesions. What is important to notice is the significant amount of shortening shown in *frame 2*, where the ostial part of the LAD is basically missing. This tip is important to bear in mind during evaluation of many ostial lesions of the LAD, where the steep caudal right anterior oblique or the steep cranial right anterior oblique may be more appropriate projections. IVUS was used to evaluate better these ostial lesions, particularly the one of the ostium of the left anterior descending. *Frame 4* shows the IVUS at the ostium of the LAD with two features: significant plaque with a residual lumen of 2.9 mm^2 and negative remodeling with the vessel diameter only 2.7 mm^2. The operator selected a 3.0×18-mm Cypher stent, which was implanted to be at the origin of the circumflex trying not to cover this vessel. In order to preserve the ostium of the circumflex, a short stent was then implanted at the ostium of the left main (Cypher 3×18 mm). The stent is deployed in the cranial RAO projection, which is usually a useful projection for viewing the origin of the left main from the aorta. The final results are shown in *frames 10* and *11*, with optimal preservation of the circumflex.

Message   The main messages of this case are as follow: use of IVUS to understand better the significance of a lesion in an ambiguous situation, the importance of learning about proper vessel size, and some angiographic tips about foreshortening and localization of ostial lesions.

4. Intermediate lesion evaluation by IVUS

Case # 11688/03

This is another example (**slides 1–4** (*frames 1–8*)) of evaluation of an intermediate lesion in the right coronary artery in a patient with clinical ischemia. Obviously, IVUS evaluation of an intermediate lesion is attempted only if there are clinical reasons for suspecting that the lesion, which angiographically does not seem critical, may be functionally critical based on symptoms or signs of ischemia. In this case, the only possible explanation for ischemia was a lesion in the right coronary artery, which did not appear angiographically critical. IVUS evaluation was performed as shown in *frame 4*, which demonstrates two elements: the lumen diameter is small, but not significantly small, with intermediate severity (3.7 mm^2), and there is important positive remodeling with vessel diameters more than 4 mm. Based on clinical presentation and on these findings, we decided to perform direct stenting with a 3.5×20-mm Taxus stent which was dilated at 16 atm. The final result is shown in *frames 7* and *8*.

Message   The main message of this case is the use of IVUS to understand better some intermediate lesions when the clinical setting suggests the presence of ischemia. Additional information is obtained by IVUS regarding appropriate vessel size and the safety of performing direct stenting.

7

Problems

Drug-eluting stent complications

1. Late-acquired stent malapposition

Case # 9676/00

As illustrated by **slides 1–3** (*runs 1–6*), this is an interesting problem, which sometimes we see with drug-eluting stents and also with non drug-eluting stents. It is a case of late stent malapposition. The baseline lesion is in the proximal part of the right coronary artery, which already at the baseline has an ectatic appearance. After Cypher-stent implantation (Cordis; 3 mm), which appears undersized, we see an optimal result in *run 2*. The 6-month angiographic and IVUS follow-up shows persistence of the good result with the IVUS. *Run 4* demonstrates that the stent is well apposed without contrast or free space behind the stent struts. The patient at this time was asymptomatic and was receiving double antiplatelet therapy. The patient returned for a scheduled 16-month angiogram and IVUS follow-up as part of the late pre-planned follow-up in a clinical study. There was an excellent angiographic result as demonstrated in *run 5*. Surprisingly, the IVUS evaluation at 16 months, as shown in *run 6*, demonstrates a large space behind the stent struts which is clearly free from any tissue as demonstrated in the direct injection during the IVUS pull back. Fortunately, this finding was not associated with any clinical event, and now, more than 2 years later, the patient continues to stay totally asymptomatic. As many studies have shown, the frequency of this problem is rare, less than 5%, and when it does occur, it does not seem to be associated with any adverse clinical event.

Message   Despite the fact that in some patients stent malapposition is found at follow-up, IVUS interrogation data from randomized DES trials have not demonstrated a higher clinical sequelae rate compared with the control group of bare-metal stents.

2. Wire-caused perforation, hematoma, slow flow and left main dissection

Case # 11374/03

This case (**slides 1–13** (*frames 1–19* and *runs 1–6*)) illustrates an attempt to reopen a chronically occluded circumflex. The operator used an Athlete intermediate wire, which caused a small perforation at the wire exit site as shown in *frame 2*. *Frame 3* illustrates a relatively localized hematoma with apparently no extension. At that time, the patient was receiving a IIb/IIIa inhibitor. Medication was immediately stopped, and owing to the fact that the hematoma appeared confined, the procedure was continued with treatment of another lesion.

The other lesion treated was a stenosis in the intermediate branch as shown in *frames 4* and *5*. A Taxus stent (3×16 mm) was deployed at this level with a good result achieved as shown in *frame 7*. Please note that the lesion did not involve the ostial segment of this vessel, and the new lesion in the proximal part of the LAD can not be related in any way to treatment of the intermediate vessel lesion. *Frames 7* and *8* illustrate a new narrowing at the ostium of the left anterior descending and in the proximal part. The most likely explanation for this new complication is the extending hematoma from the circumflex, which is now compressing the LAD. *Frame 9* shows the hematoma located near the new lesion with a Taxus stent which was promptly advanced in order to establish immediate patency. *Frame 10* shows the ostium of the LAD now well patent.

In order to seal the hematoma, the next step was to implant a PTFE-covered stent over the proximal part of the circumflex where the perforation occurred. *Frames 11* and *13* show deployment of this stent. The final result is presented in *runs 1* and *2*, which now show slow flow at the level of the LAD. This event was most probably due to protrusion of the stent in the distal left main with the left anterior descending being compromised. The operator was able to advance a wire and to perform intravascular ultrasound, which shows (*frame 14* and *run 3*) a small ostium of the LAD with the struts of the PTFE-covered stent protruding in this vessel.

The next step was to advance a balloon at this level and to perform a kissing balloon inflation in the intermediate and in the LAD; the cross-sectional area in the left anterior descending improved from 1.6 to 7.6 mm^2 as shown in *run 4*. The result following inflation of the LAD and intermediate is shown in *frames 16* and *17*. Unfortunately, this never-ending series of complications is now with a new dissection in the proximal part of the left main. This problem was treated with implantation of a Taxus stent (3.5 mm), which was post-dilated with a 4-mm balloon, and the final result is demonstrated in *runs 5* and *6*.

Message   There are several messages that can be learned from this case. The most important message is not to lose courage, to remain calm and to treat each complication one after the other. The second message is to try to stay away from IIb/IIIa while performing total occlusion treatment. As a matter of fact, the operator did not plan to reopen the circumflex initially, and this was a change in strategy when we had already planned to treat the native vessels with IIb/IIIa pretreatment. The third element to keep in mind is always to place a wire when positioning a stent at the ostium of another branch, sometimes not only a wire but also to park a balloon at that level in case the stent will protrude too much. The presence of the balloon can also help to evaluate the exact positioning of the stent. This message is even more important when the stent used is a PTFE-covered stent.

3. Wire-caused perforation with delayed tamponade

Case # 11881/04

This case (slides 1–12 (*frames 1–17* and *runs 1–9*)) illustrates stenting of the distal left main and of the proximal LAD in a patient with calcific disease. The procedure was first started with pre-dilatation using a 3-mm balloon and then a cutting balloon in order to prepare the vessel. The next step was the advancement of a 3.5×33-mm Cypher stent. Please note the presence of a balloon pump, which is very frequently used when treating unprotected left main coronary arteries. Unfortunately, the Cypher stent could not be advanced in the more distal part of the lesion with the goal of covering entirely the diseased segment. The operator deployed the stent more proximally because it appears sufficiently advanced to treat the left main and the proximal LAD. Following stent deployment, there was a small dissection in the left anterior descending which clearly needed to be treated. The operator pre-dilated this area with a high-pressure balloon (20 atm) and inserted a second wire in order to gain more support. Unfortunately, various maneuvers were unsuccessful in advancing a stent in this location, and maneuvering the wire in order to gain support caused a distal perforation with the tip of the wire. The wire involved in this perforation was a Whisper wire (Guidant). *Frame 8* and *run 1* show the perforation at the apex of the left ventricle. The perforation appeared relatively stable and the procedure was stopped.

About 2 h later the patient experienced severe hypotension with clinical signs of tamponade and underwent emergency pericardiocentesis; a further angiogram did not demonstrate increased bleeding in the apex, but there was clear persistence of dye extravasation. Despite reversal of heparin with protamine, the pigtail catheter continued to drain blood from the pericardium. The operator decided to occlude the distal LAD with polyvinyl alcohol particles distally injected with a Transit catheter. These particles were injected as shown in *run 3*, which demonstrates the Transit advanced very distally in the left anterior descending. *Run 4* demonstrates an injection immediately after the particle administration in the distal LAD, with *frame 9* showing a distal LAD occlusion. No more blood was drained from the pericardium. Unfortunately, following this maneuver, there is the appearance of gross thrombus in the proximal left anterior descending, distal left main and proximal part of the intermediate branch. The patient became again unstable, and immediate counterpulsation had to be restarted. An aspiration catheter was advanced in the proximal LAD and distal left main and balloon angioplasty was performed following re-wiring of the left anterior descending and of the intermediate branch.

Fortunately, the situation became stable with regained patency. At this time, heparin was also administered due to the fact that the distal perforation appeared sealed. The patient remained on balloon counterpulsation overnight, and the control angiogram 24 h later showed good patency of the left main and proximal LAD, and no distal leaking with the occlusion of the peri-apical left anterior descending. At this time, a new attempt was made to cover the mid LAD lesions. The area was pre-dilated again with balloon angioplasty, with cutting balloon, and then a Taxus stent (3 × 12 mm) was first advanced but did not reach the distal part of the lesion, and was then deployed more proximally but covering one segment of the diseased artery.

The final segment was successfully covered with a very short Cypher stent as demonstrated in *frame 17*. Runs *8* and *9* demonstrate the final result with good flow and full coverage of the left anterior descending in the proximal and mid part.

4. LIMA perforation

Case # 10780/02

Case # 10780/02 is illustrated by **slides 1–5** (*frames 1–9* and *run 1*). The case illustrates a patient with a left mammary artery anastomosed to an intermediate branch as shown in *frame 2*. There is diffuse narrowing in the distal segment of the mammary at the site of the anastomosis and distally in the native intermediate branch. The vessel was dilated with a 2.0-mm balloon as shown in *frame 3* and *4*, with the result shown in *frame 5*. The next step was implantation of a Cypher stent (2.5 × 33 mm) positioned across the anastomotic site with half of the stent protruding in the mammary and half in the intermediate branch. The stent was inflated at 18 atm. Following deployment, there was a perforation involving mainly the mammary artery. The next step in such a case would usually be to consider a PTFE-covered stent, but due to tortuousity in the mammary artery, this procedure may be fairly complex. The operator decided to perform prolonged balloon inflation following protamine injection, and the perforation was successfully sealed as shown in *frame 9*.

Message   Apart from trying to position a PTFE-covered stent, the options when dealing with a perforation are to do a prolonged balloon inflation or to position a bare-metal stent; sometimes bare-metal stents may help, and on other occasions positioning a bare-metal stent may facilitate the advancement of a PTFE-covered stent.

5. Wire-caused perforation while attempting to re-open chronic total occlusion

Case # 11658/02

This case (**slides 1–5** (*frames 1–10*)) demonstrates treatment of a patient with chronic renal failure and severe coronary artery disease with occlusion of the mid left anterior descending and the distal intermediate branch. *Frames 1* and *2* show the baseline disease in the left coronary system. An attempt was made to re-open the left anterior descending; the wire was advanced distally but most probably created an exit from the LAD as demonstrated by the arrows in *frame 3*. The wire was repositioned more proximally, and an angiogram did not demonstrate any dye extravasation. *Frame 6* shows no signs of distal dye extravasation in the left anterior descending. The vessel was treated in its proximal and mid part with two Taxus stents as demonstrated in *frames 7* and *8*. *Frames 9* and *10* show the absence of dye extravasation in the final angiogram, but unfortunately the patient developed late tamponade requiring pericardiocentesis.

Message It is rare, but possible, that a hydrophilic wire will cause a perforation without clear angiographic evidence of dye extravasation, and the only clinical manifestation could be a delayed tamponade.

6. Intra-procedural stent thrombosis with DES

Case # 10766/02

This is a case of intraprocedural stent thrombosis (**slide 1** and **slides 2–4** (*frame 1* and *runs 1–5*)). The patient was treated in the mid left anterior descending with a 33-mm Cypher stent successfully positioned in a lesion in this vessel. Owing to some chest pain occurring the day after admission, the patient was re-evaluated with a new angiogram 3 days following the index procedure. This angiogram demonstrated a small residual dissection in the distal part of the left anterior descending just distally to the previously positioned stent. *Frame 1* (see arrow) illustrates the small distal dissection. The operator elected to implant a short Cypher stent, which was very easily advanced in the distal LAD. Immediately after inflation of the stent and following removal of the wire, the patient experienced severe chest pain, and an immediate injection showed no distal flow in the distal part of the LAD and a filling defect in the proximal part, which immediately progressed into extensive thrombosis of the left main and of the circumflex. A wire was re-advanced, and following supportive measures with adrenaline and additional heparin and IIb/IIIa administration, patency was re-established at the level of all major epicardial vessels in the left system. Unfortunately, the patient did not reach a stable hemodynamic condition despite balloon counterpulsation. An emergency surgical revascularization was unsuccessful, and the patient expired following the surgical procedure.

Message This case illustrates a very rare but nevertheless reported phenomenon of intra-procedural stent thrombosis with drug-eluting stents. The cause of this event is unclear. The patient appeared adequately anticoagulated with heparin, and in a multivariate analysis the stent length was most probably the most important predisposing cause rather than the type of stent *per se*.

7. Vessel perforation with difficulties in advancing a PTFE-covered stent

Case # HSR 35897

Case # HSR 35897 is illustrated by **slides 1–8** (*frames 1–12* and *runs 1–6*). *Frame 1* illustrates a lesion in an intermediate branch in a patient with prior by-pass surgery. The operator assumed that the vessel was fibrotic on the evidence that vessels in patients with prior by-pass surgery are frequently calcified and difficult to dilate; the operator elected to use a cutting balloon (3 mm). The result was a perforation with a coronary rupture as illustrated in *run 1* and *frame 3*. This complication is rare but can occur with a cutting balloon, particularly if it is oversized and sometimes if it is inflated at the site of a curve as in this case. Following the perforation and after unsuccessful prolonged balloon inflation (as shown in *frame 4*) and due to persistence of leakage as demonstrated in *run 2*, an attempt was made to advance a PTFE-covered stent as shown in *frame 5*. Unfortunately, the covered stent could not be implanted distally enough to cover the perforation, and the leakage persisted as shown in *run 3*. The leakage is better demonstrated in *frame 6* (see arrow). A second PTFE-covered stent could not be successfully advanced at the level of the perforation, as demonstrated in *run 4*. A different approach was then chosen, which involved placing several noncovered stents. This approach is utilized sometimes in an attempt to seal the perforation by compressing flaps of dissection and compacting the tissues. Some operators have reported successful results using this strategy. *Frames 7–9* demonstrate implantation of three bare-metal stents, with *run 5* showing the result following implantation of these multiple bare-metal stents. Despite a reduction in leakage, there is still extravasation of contrast from the artery. At this point, a final attempt was made to advance a 3-mm covered stent; most probably due to the better opening and reshaping of the vessel by the bare-metal stents, the PTFE-covered stent could be advanced and positioned correctly. Following deployment of the PTFE-covered stent shown in *frame 11*, *run 6* shows complete sealing of the leakage.

Message   Two messages can be learned from this case. The first one is that use of the cutting balloon is important and helpful, but it is not always free from the risk of perforation, particularly in an angulated lesion and if oversized, as in this case. The second message is that the use of bare-metal stents can sometimes be of help in a perforation – if not to close the perforation to allow better advancement of a PTFE-covered stent. As a general rule, a proximal stent does not facilitate advancement of a stent more distally, but sometimes it does, particularly when there is no other solution available.

8. Managing a perforation

Case # 11281/03

This case (**slides 1–6** (*frames 1–5* and *runs 1–8*)) illustrates a complication which can occur with the deployment of any type of stent – drug-eluting or non drug-eluting. The case concerns an ostial lesion of the circumflex involving a bifurcation of the obtuse marginal branch with a filling defect, suggestive of calcification, in a patient with stable angina. The procedure was initiated with rotational atherectomy utilizing a somewhat conservative approach: a burr of 1.75 mm in diameter as shown in *frame 1*. Following rotablation, which was uneventful, a Bx Velocity Hepacoat stent (Cordis) (3.0×8 mm) was implanted at the ostium of the circumflex. During stent implantation, the occurrence of a Type III perforation (as shown in *run 3*) became apparent. It is not unusual for the consequences of a perforation, most probably triggered by rotational atherectomy, to become manifest during post-dilatation or during stent implantation.

   At this point, the only option was to exclude the vessel from which the perforation was coming – the distal circumflex. A PTFE-covered stent fortunately was advanced into the obtuse marginal branch, and it was able to seal the perforation. The next step was to dilate the new lesion in the ostial LAD, most probably caused by plaque shift. *Frame 3*, at the time of stent deployment, shows a compromise of the ostium of the LAD. A stent was positioned at this level: Hepacoat 3.5×18 mm, with a good result. It is interesting to see in *runs 5* and *6* that the distal circumflex maintains some patency. The 1-month follow-up demonstrated in *runs 7* and *8* shows excellent patency of the stent in the LAD and of the PTFE-covered stent with closure of the proximal circumflex. Collaterals are now coming from the distal obtuse marginal branch and probably from the left anterior descending.

Message   The main message of this case is that perforations can occur even at the time of dilatation with a balloon following rotational atherectomy. The availability of PTFE-covered stents has to be maintained in every cardiac catheterization laboratory. Sealing of a perforation sometimes may require occlusion of a side branch that originates from the site of the perforation. These are conditions in which the most severe problem needs to be addressed at the price of some known complications.

Complications with drug-eluting stents: my worst nightmares

Matthew J Price MD, *Paul S Teirstein* MD

Case 1

A 54-year-old male with a history of Cypher stenting of the right coronary artery presented for staged intervention of the left circumflex artery prior to high-risk noncardiac surgery (slides 1–5 (*frames 1–8*)).

Selective left coronary angiography through an 8-Fr guide confirmed the presence of a significant stenosis in a large first obtuse marginal. This lesion spanned a branch vessel of moderate caliber with mild disease at its ostium (slide 1, *frame 1*).

Direct stenting of the lesion was performed with a 2.5×13-mm Cypher stent (Cordis) deployed at 18 atm. Left coronary angiography demonstrated an excellent angiographic result within the obtuse marginal, but significant compromise of the ostium of the branch vessel was apparent (slide 1, *frame 2*).

A Pilot 150 wire (Guidant) was advanced through the stent struts, and the ostium of the side branch was dilated with a 2.5×12-mm Maverick balloon (Boston Scientific). Subsequent angiography demonstrated TIMI II flow with a type C dissection in the side branch (slide 2, *frame 3*).

To treat the dissection, an attempt was made to stent the side-branch ostium. However, a 2.5×18-mm Cypher stent could not be advanced across the stent strut, and thus further pre-dilatation of the side-branch ostium was performed with a 2.75×9-mm Maverick balloon. With significant difficulty that required deep intubation of the guide within the left main coronary artery, the 2.5×18-mm Cypher stent was successfully advanced into the side branch and was deployed using a kissing balloon inflation with a 2.5×9-mm Maverick balloon within the main, obtuse marginal branch (slide 2, *frame 4*).

Subsequent coronary angiography demonstrated a dissection of the left main coronary artery extending into the left anterior descending (LAD) and circumflex arteries (slide 3, *frame 5*). A second wire was advanced into the distal LAD, and intra-aortic balloon counterpulsation was initiated. Additional Cypher stents to treat the dissection could not be advanced into the LAD nor into the proximal left circumflex (LCX) – the latter because the distal stent edge could not cross the proximal edge of the previously placed stent. Thus, extensive balloon dilatation of these areas was performed. Two Cypher stents were then positioned within the left main in a double-barrel fashion: a 3.0×33-mm Cypher stent extending into the LAD and a 3.0×18-mm Cypher stent extending into the LCX. The stents were simultaneously deployed at 18 atm (slide 3, *frame 6*). Angiography demonstrated TIMI 3 flow with containment of the dissection (slide 4, *frame 7*).

Surveillance angiography was performed 3 months later (slide 5, *frames 8a, 8b*). This demonstrated no in-stent restenosis within the left main, the left anterior descending, or the left circumflex arteries.

Case 2

This case concerns a 78-year-old male with a history of coronary artery disease who presented with chest discomfort (slides 6–9 (*frames 9–13*)). Clinical examination and chest roentgenography were consistent with pulmonary edema. Electrocardiography showed dynamic ST depression in the precordial leads, and cardiac enzymes were negative. Given his presentation consistent with severe ongoing ischemia, he was referred for coronary angiography.

Selective left coronary angiography demonstrated a critical stenosis within the mid-portion of the left main coronary artery and significant disease within the left anterior descending artery (slide 6, *frame 9*). The right coronary artery was dominant, with significant stenoses distally and within the proximal posterolateral branch (not shown). While discussing the option of cardiac surgery with the patient's family, the patient developed ventricular tachycardia and then ventricular fibrillation. Defibrillation was successful but now the patient was in electro-mechanical disassociation without ventricular contractions. Selective left coronary angiography was performed with a guide-catheter during cardiopulmonary resuscitation, revealing acute closure of the left main coronary artery (slide 6, *frame 10*). Flow was re-established after dilatation of the left main and left anterior descending arteries with a 3.25×15-mm Quantum Maverick balloon (slide 7, *frame 11*). Ventricular contractions then resumed and chest compressions were discontinued. Two 3.0×23-mm cypher stents were then deployed within the mid LAD, followed by a 3.5×13-mm Cypher stent within the left main coronary artery (slide 7, *frame 12a*, slide 8, *frames 12b, 12c*). The next day, transthoracic echocardiography showed normal left ventricular function. The patient returned 3 months later for percutaneous intervention of the right coronary artery. Left coronary angiography revealed no in-stent restenosis within the left main or left anterior descending arteries (slide 9, *frame 13*).

DISCUSSION

These two cases raise three important issues regarding the use of Cypher stents: (a) the treatment of bifurcational lesions, (b) common scenarios which require adequate pre-dilatation, and (c) left main coronary artery stenting.

Bifurcational lesions and Cypher stents

Multiple approaches to bifurcational lesions have been proposed. Stenting across the side branch with provisional angioplasty or stenting has been shown to be effective. However, significant procedural morbidity may occasionally occur in the event of side-branch compromise when a wire, balloon, or stent can not cross through the stent struts into the side-branch lumen. Indeed, side-branch compromise and unsuccessful stent implantation may occur in nearly 10% of cases.[1] This may be prevented by establishing access to both lumens intially and then stenting both branches. Although nonrandomized observational studies have not demonstrated an advantage to bare-metal stenting of the side branch compared with balloon angioplasty alone, the antiproliferative effects of drug-eluting stents may reduce the incidence of restenosis and thereby improve clinical outcomes.

A randomized study to test this hypothesis was recently performed.[2] 'True' bifurcational lesions with greater than 50% stenoses in both the main branch and the ostium of the side branch were randomized to treatment with either Cypher stenting of both branches or stenting of the main branch with angioplasty of the side branch. T-stenting was the technique used in 95% of the lesions treated with two stents. Of the patients randomized to angioplasty of the side branch, 51% crossed over to the stent group because of suboptimal angiographic results. Analysis was performed according to the actual treatment received. Procedural success was significantly better in the double-stenting group (93.6% vs. 77.3%), but binary restenosis at the 6-month follow-up was no different (double stenting 28.0%, side-branch angioplasty 18.7%, $p = 0.53$). Restenosis in both groups occurred predominantly at the ostium of the side-branch. Intravascular ultrasound evaluation was performed in four of the cases of ostial side-branch in-stent restenosis; in three, incomplete stent coverage was observed. Techniques such as 'crush' or 'double barrel' (also known as 'V') stenting that ensure full stent coverage of both limbs of the bifurcation may further reduce in-stent restenosis of the ostium of the side branch.

In 20 patients with bifurcational lesions treated by crush stenting, there was 100% angiographic success, three in-hospital adverse cardiac events (one Q-wave MI, one non-Q-wave MI, and one target-lesion revascularization due to distal dissection) and no events over a mean of 1.5 months of clinical follow-up.[3] Further study is needed to determine whether full stent coverage of the bifurcation will prevent ostial-branch restenosis. Moreover, it must be determined whether the efficacy and safety profile of the Cypher stent will be affected by the altered pharmacokinetics of sirolimus delivery that may result from stent strut distortion and the presence of multiple stent layers.

Inability to deliver additional stents

The inability to advance a second stent across the proximal edge of an initially deployed stent is a common scenario. This is more likely to occur if the initial stent was deployed at a relatively low pressure because the distal edge of the second stent or its delivery system may 'catch' on the proximal edge of the initially deployed stent. Often the need for an additional stent is recognized only after the deployment of the first. However, if the need for additional stenting is recognized while the initial stent balloon is still in place, one can slightly withdraw the stent balloon and perform an additional inflation at a higher pressure to improve proximal stent expansion. Alternatively, post-dilatation of the proximal edge can be carefully performed with a second balloon. A Wiggle wire (Guidant) may also be helpful in this situation. One caveat unique to drug-eluting stenting is the need to cover all injured areas with stent; thus post-dilation at the proximal stent edge should not be performed unless additional stenting is planned.

Cypher stents for 'bailout' of left main dissection
or acute myocardial infarction

The SIRIUS study did not include patients with left main lesions, and the efficacy of left main intervention with Cypher stents has not yet been well studied. One case series of 31 patients who underwent PCI of the left main with Cypher stents demonstrated excellent clinical outcomes over 5 months of follow-up.[4] Angiographic follow-up was not performed. Twenty of these patients had unprotected left main coronary arteries. Nine patients underwent 'bailout' stenting for left main dissection, similar to the patient described in case 1. Of these, there were no in-hospital or post-discharge events, except for one patient who underwent subsequent coronary bypass surgery during the index hospitalization.

Of 17 patients who underwent left main stenting electively (7 unprotected), there was one in-hospital myocardial infarction, one death, and no post-discharge events. Patients who underwent Cypher stenting of the left main coronary artery for acute myocardial infarction did not have very successful outcomes: three out of five patients died in hospital. Fortunately, the patient in case 2 occluded his left main coronary artery in the cardiac catheterization laboratory, and antegrade flow was quickly re-established while cardiopulmonary resuscitation was performed; his left ventricular function was preserved, and he was doing well at the 3-month follow-up. It is not known whether the large diameter of the left main, the distortion of the stent strut architecture by the crush technique, or the neocarina formed by the double-barrel technique may compromise the anti-restenotic efficacy or safety profile of the Cypher stent. Indefinite clopidogrel therapy and surveillance angiography 2–3 months after the index procedure is recommended. If shown to be effective in preventing in-stent restenosis, Cypher stenting of the left main coronary artery would represent an exciting development in the percutaneous treatment of patients with severe coronary artery disease.

REFERENCES

1. Pan M, Suarez de Lezo J, Medina A, et al. A stepwise strategy for the stent treatment of bifurcated coronary lesions. Catheter Cardiovasc Interv 2002; 55: 50–7
2. Colombo A, Moses JW, Morice MC, et al. Randomized study to evaluate sirolimus-eluting stents implanted at coronary bifurcation lesions. Circulation 2004; 23: 23

3. Colombo A, Stankovic G, Orlic D, et al. Modified T-stenting technique with crushing for bifurcation lesions: immediate results and 30-day outcome. Catheter Cardiovasc Interv 2003; 60: 145–51
4. Arampatzis CA, Lemos PA, Tanabe K, et al. Effectiveness of sirolimus-eluting stent for treatment of left main coronary artery disease. Am J Cardiol 2003; 92: 327–9

Stent thrombosis after Cypher and Taxus stent implantation

Antonio Colombo MD, *Ioannis Iakovou* MD

Despite the major improvements of antiplatelet therapy, thrombotic events remain the primary cause of death after percutaneous coronary interventions (PCI).[1,2] Recently, polymer-based paclitaxel-eluting stents (PES) (Taxus, Boston Scientific) and sirolimus-eluting stents (SES) (Cypher, Cordis) have been shown to reduce neointimal hyperplasia and risk of restenosis.[3–5] Cases of subacute thrombosis in drug-eluting stents (DES) have been recently scrutinized, and the US FDA has released an advisory notice informing physicians about adverse events, and more specifically subacute thrombosis (SAT) associated with the sirolimus-eluting stents (SES) Cypher.[6] There is a particular need to evaluate the incidence of these adverse events in unselected patients and lesions representing the 'real-world' patient population.

We evaluated the incidence of stent thrombosis after sirolimus-eluting stent and paclitaxel-eluting stent implantation in unselected lesions: 1769 consecutive patients who underwent SES (921 patients, 1725 lesions, 1953 stents) or PES (848 patients, 1159 lesions, 1448 stents) implantation in 3 institutions (Centro Cuore Columbus and San Raffaele Hospital, Milan, Italy and Department of Cardiology, Klinikum Siegburg Rhein-Sieg GmbH, Siegburg, Germany) were identified. All patients were pretreated with ticlopidine or clopidogrel and aspirin; a loading dose of 300 mg of clopidogrel was given to those who were not pretreated. Aspirin was continued indefinitely and clopidogrel or ticlopidine for at least 3 months following SES implantation and for at least 6 months following PES implantation. Stent implantation methods have been described previously.[7] All stents were implanted with high-pressure final balloon dilatation in an attempt to cover fully the angiographic lesion with the stent. Glycoprotein IIb/IIIa inhibitors were administered at the operators' discretion.

Stent thrombosis definitions

Stent thrombosis definitions included any of the following: angiographic documentation of stent occlusion or filling defects inside the stent in the first month following stenting, unexplained sudden death without concomitant demonstration of patency of the stent, myocardial infarction in the area of the implanted stent, or

Table 1   Baseline clinical and angiographic characteristics

	SES	PES	p
Patient characteristics			
Patients (n)	921	848	
Male gender (%)	77	78	0.9
Age (years)	61 ± 10	61 ± 11	0.9
Unstable angina (%)	28	27	0.6
Diabetes (%)	24	25	0.6
Hypertension (%)	62	59	0.2
Hypercholesterolemia (%)	69	62	0.001
Family history of coronary artery disease (%)	35	43	0.0005
Current smoking (%)	16	18	0.2
Previous myocardial infarction (%)	45	49	0.09
Previous percutaneous coronary intervention (%)	52	44	0.0007
Previous bypass surgery (%)	22	29	0.0007
Multivessel disease (%)	89	87	0.2
Left ventricular ejection fraction (%)	53 ± 9	53 ± 10	0.1
Lesion characteristics			
Lesions (n)	1725	1159	
Vessels treated			
Left anterior descending artery (%)	41	43	0.3
Left circumflex (%)	25	21	0.01
Right coronary artery (%)	31	33	0.3
Saphenous vein graft (%)	2	2.3	0.6
Arterial graft (%)	0.9	0.3	0.6
Ostial location (%)	16	12	0.002
Proximal location (%)	37	39	0.3
B2 or C lesions (%)	79	78	0.5
Total occlusion (%)	14	15	0.9
Bifurcation (%)	28	25	0.07
Calcium (%)	10	19	<0.0001
Thrombus (%)	1.4	2	0.2
Preintervention TIMI 3 (%)	82	85	0.03

Values are presented as numbers (relative percentages) or mean ± standard deviation. PES, paclitaxel-eluting stents; SES, sirolimus-eluting stents; TIMI, thrombolysis in myocardial infarction

urgent target-lesion revascularization (TLR).[8] Stent thrombosis cases were categorized according to the timing of the above-mentioned events into acute (AT, <24 h), subacute (SAT, >24 h up to 30 days) and late (LST, >30 days).

Baseline clinical and angiographic characteristics

Patient baseline clinical and angiographic characteristics are shown in Table 1. Family history of coronary artery disease and by-pass surgery were more frequent in the SES group, and hypercholesterolemia and previous PCI more common in the PES group. There were no other statistically significant differences regarding the baseline clinical characteristics. Left circumflex, ostial lesions, and bifurcations were more frequently found in the SES group; conversely, calcified lesions and preintervention TIMI 3 flow were more frequent in the PES group.

In-hospital outcome and acute stent thrombosis

All stents were deployed successfully. There were no statistically significant differences between the two stent groups regarding the procedural characteristics apart from a larger maximum balloon diameter in the PES group, as shown in Table 2. However, PES-treated lesions had significantly shorter length, and larger post-procedural RVD and MLD. There were no significant differences between the two groups regarding the procedural complications and the in-hospital outcome. Acute stent thrombosis occurred in four patients in the SES group and three patients in the PES group (0.4% vs. 0.3%, $p = 0.9$).

Thirty-day clinical outcome and subacute stent thrombosis

Thirty-day follow-up was available in all patients and is shown in Table 3. There were no statistical significant differences regarding death, stroke, Q-wave myocardial infarction, TLR, and cumulative major adverse cardiac event (MACE). The overall incidence of SAT was 0.6% occurring in three patients after SES implantation and in eight patients after PES implantation (0.3% vs. 0.9%, $p = 0.2$). The itemized clinical and procedural characteristics of patients with subacute thrombosis are presented in Table 4. One of the three, and seven of the eight SAT cases of the SES and PES groups, respectively, occurred within 1 week post-procedure.

The first case of SAT in the SES group refers to a patient previously treated with intracoronary brachytherapy and presenting as an acute MI. This patient was treated initially with thrombolysis and subsequently underwent early PCI and bypass surgery. Patient number 2 with SAT in the SES group had discontinued his antiplatelet medication 10 days before the event, and he was treated with thrombolysis. The third patient (number 3), with a history of chronic renal failure, developed contrast-induced nephropathy and died 15 days post-procedure after cardiac arrest. Out of the eight patients who sustained SAT following PES implantation, two died suddenly, one discontinued antiplatelet therapy prematurely, and two had bifurcational stenting with two or more stents implanted.

Late stent thrombosis

At follow-up (mean: 9.6±4.3 months for SES and 7.6±3.2 months for PES), LST occurred in four (0.4%) patients in the SES group and in four (0.4%) patients in the

Table 2   Procedural data and in-hospital outcome

	SES	PES	p
Procedural characteristics			
Procedures (n)	921	848	
Maximum balloon diameter (mm)	2.95±0.48	3.06±0.57	<0.0001
Maximum balloon inflation (atm)	16.4±3.2	16.6±3.3	0.2
Stent length per lesion (mm)	27.71±13.21	27.22±13.49	0.4
Stents per lesion	1.13±0.40	1.13±0.41	1.0
Glycoprotein IIb/IIIa inhibitors (%)	42	40	0.4
Procedural complications			
Intra-aortic balloon pump, n (%)	6 (0.6)	2 (0.2)	0.3
Acute stent thrombosis, n (%)	5 (0.5)	3 (0.3)	0.8
TIMI 0–2, n (%)	5 (0.5)	2 (0.2)	0.5
Dissection after stent, n (%)	9 (1.0)	3 (0.3)	0.2
Perforation, n (%)	3 (0.3)	8 (0.9)	0.1
Quantitative coronary angiography			
Lesions (n)	1725	1159	
Preintervention			
RVD (mm)	2.62±0.60	2.59±0.64	0.2
MLD (mm)	0.86±0.53	0.89±0.51	0.1
DS (%)	67±17	66±17	0.2
Lesion length (mm)	18.57±14.72	16.68±12.14	<0.001
Postintervention			
RVD (mm)	3.01±0.52	3.14±0.65	<0.001
MLD (mm)	2.64±0.51	2.75±0.62	<0.001
DS (%)	12±8	12±9	1.0
In-hospital outcome			
Death, n (%)	1 (0.1)	3 (0.3)*	0.6
Q-wave myocardial infarction, n (%)	1 (0.1)	2 (0.2)	0.9
Non-Q-wave myocardial infarction, n (%)	114 (12)	105 (12)	1.0
Stroke, n (%)	0	0	0
Emergency bypass surgery, n (%)	1 (0.1)	0	0.9
Repeat PCI, n (%)	2 (0.2)	1 (0.1)	0.9
Angiographic success (%)	100	100	

*Two deaths due to cardiogenic shock unrelated to stent implantation. Values are presented as numbers (relative percentages) or mean±standard deviation. DS, diameter stenosis; MLD, minimal lumen diameter; RVD, reference vessel diameter; TIMI, thrombolysis in myocardial infarction

PES group ($p = 0.8$). One patient of the SES group who suffered late thrombosis had discontinued antiplatelet therapy (including aspirin) 10 days before the event (38 days post-stenting). Overall, there were 26 cases (1.47%) of stent thrombosis in

Table 3   Thirty-day out of hospital clinical outcome

Variable	SES	PES	p
Patients (*n*)	921	848	
Death, *n* (%)	2 (0.2)*	5 (0.6)[†]	0.4
Stroke, *n* (%)	1 (0.1)*	0	0.9
Q-wave myocardial infarction, *n* (%)	2 (0.2)	6 (0.7)	0.2
Target-lesion revascularization, *n* (%)	1 (0.1)	5 (0.6)	0.1
Subacute stent thrombosis, *n* (%)	3 (0.3)	8 (0.9)	0.1
Cumulative MACE, *n* (%)[‡]	3 (0.3)	8 (0.9)	0.1

*One patient with cerebrovascular accident resulting in non-cardiac death
[†]One death due to cardiogenic shock unrelated to stent implantation
[‡]Patients with more than one event are counted as one

the 1769 patients treated with DES, with no difference between patients treated with SES or PES (1.2% for SES and 1.8% for PES, $p = 0.9$) as shown in Table 5.

Predictors of thrombosis

Stent length was identified as a predictor of both acute (Figure 1) (OR = 1.04; 95% CI, 1.01 to 1.10 with bootstrap Gong's selection 64%) and subacute thrombosis (Figure 2) (OR = 1.03; 95% CI, 1.02 to 1.06 with bootstrap Gong's selection 79%), while B2 or C type lesion was a predictor of subacute thrombosis (OR = 1.37; 95% CI, 1.10 to 1.74 with bootstrap Gong's selection 10%). No predictors were identified regarding LST (Figure 3). Stent length (OR = 1.02; 95% CI, 1.009 to 1.04 with bootstrap Gong's selection 58%) and B2 and C type lesion (OR = 1.20; 95% CI, 1.04 to 1.48 with bootstrap Gong's selection 17%) were identified as predictors of any stent thrombosis, as shown in Figure 4.

FINDINGS

The main finding of the present study is that in patients with unselected lesions treated with the two types of DES currently available on the market, the incidence of any stent thrombosis at mean follow-up of 9 months for SES and 7 months for PES is 1.47%. There were no statistically significant differences regarding the combined incidence of stent thrombosis (acute, subacute, and late) between the two type of stents. Lesion length and B2 or C type lesion were identified as predictors of thrombotic events after DES implantation.

Stent thrombosis is regarded as a mutlifactorial process consisting of device-related (stent thrombogenicity), patient or lesion, and procedure-related factors.[9] In our study, stent length and B2 or C type lesion were identified as predictors of thrombosis after DES implantation. These results are in accordance with previous

Table 4 Itemized clinical and procedural characteristics of patients with subacute thrombosis

No.	Age, gender	Restenosis	PCI indication	Artery stented	Stent type	No. of stents	Total stent length (mm)	Presentation	Outcome
1	42, M	Yes	UA	LAD	Cypher	3	99	AMI 6 days post-procedure	Thrombolysis → PCI → CABG (3 months post-procedure)
2	80, M*	No	UA	LAD, diagonal bifurcation	Cypher	4	117	AMI 26 days post-procedure	Thrombolysis
3	75, M	No	UA	LAD	Cypher	3	84	Cardiac arrest and death 15 days post-procedure	–
4	69, M	No	SA	LCX,LM, LAD bifurcation	Taxus	1	32	AMI 25 days post-procedure	Thrombolysis → PCI
5	70, M	Yes	SA	Protected LM, LCX	Taxus	3	52	AMI 3 days post-procedure	Thrombolysis → PCI → death (3 months post-procedure)
6	67, M	No	UA	Protected LM, LAD	Taxus	3	60	AMI 4 days post-procedure	PCI death 4 days post-procedure
7	81, M	No	SA	LM	Taxus	2	32	Death 4 days post-procedure	–
8	72, M	No	UA	LAD, D1 bifurcation	Taxus	2	52	AMI 4 days post-procedure	Unsuccesfull attempt to recanalize D1
9	48, M	No	UA	LAD	Taxus	1	24	AMI 4 days post-procedure	Thrombolysis → angiographic documentation
10	72, M	No	UA	LCX	Taxus	3	64	AMI 4 days post-procedure	Primary PCI → UA 2 days post-procedure → PCI
11	67, M	No	SA	LM	Taxus	2	40	Death 6 days post-procedure	–

*Patient discontinued antiplatelet therapy 1 week prior to event

AMI, acute myocardial infarction; LAD, left anterior descending; LCX, left circumflex; LM, left main; SA, stable angina; UA, unstable angina; CABG; coronary artery bypass graft

Table 5 Incidence of stent thrombosis

Variable	SES	PES	p value
Patients (*n*)	921	848	
Acute stent thrombosis, *n* (%)	4 (0.4)	3 (0.3)	0.9
Subacute stent thrombosis, *n* (%)	3 (0.3)*†	8 (0.9)§‖	0.2
Late stent thrombosis, *n* (%)	4 (0.4)‡	4 (0.4)	0.8
Total stent thrombosis, *n* (%)	11 (1.2)	15 (1.8)	0.4

*One patient with antiplatelet therapy discontinuation
†One patient with chronic renal failure and death after cardiac arrest
‡One patient with aspirin discontinuation
§One patient with clopidogrel discontinuation one day prior to the event
‖One patient with two events; PES, paclitaxel-eluting stents; SES, sirolimus-eluting stents

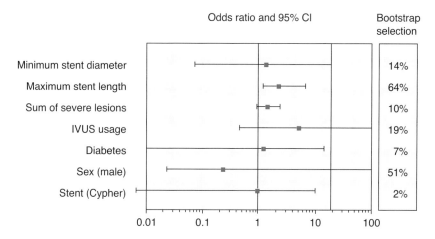

Figure 1 Univariate predictors of acute stent thrombosis by bootstrap analysis

studies with bare-metal stents which identified pre-intervention lesion characteristics and stent length as significant risk factors of stent thrombosis.[10]

In the present study, 24 out of the 26 cases of DES thrombosis occurred in B2 or C type lesions. It is interesting to note, that all 11 cases of SAT were B2 or C type lesions. Moreover, one of the SES patients with SAT had prior intracoronary beta radiation treatment at the target vessel. It has been suggested that the damage to the endothelial lining of capillaries, arterioles, and arteries that occurs after radiation exposure is associated with increased thrombogenicity.[11] Patient demographics and, in particular, old age and unstable angina have been implicated with stent thrombosis.[12,13] In our study, 6 out of the 11 patients with SAT were older than 70 years. Similarly, seven of these patients had unstable angina, and six were diabetics.

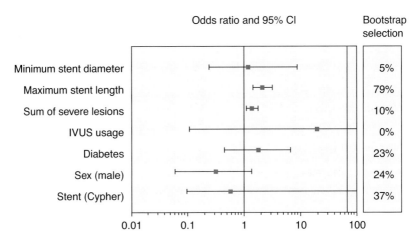

Figure 2   Univariate predictors of subacute stent thrombosis by bootstrap analysis

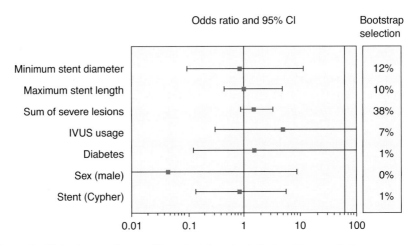

Figure 3   Univariate predictors of late stent thrombosis by bootstrap analysis

Post-procedural lesion characteristics have also been associated with SAT. It must be noted that in all cases of SAT, the immediate angiographic result was acceptable apart from two cases with residual lesions distally to the stent (both in the PES group). It has recently been suggested that inadequate post-procedure lumen dimensions, alone or in combination with other procedurally related abnormal lesion morphologies, contribute to this phenomenon.[8,10,14] Furthermore, we have previously shown that factors that may predispose to SAT in bare-metal stents are

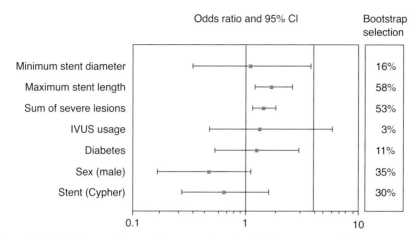

Figure 4   Univariate predictors of any stent thrombosis by bootstrap analysis

low ejection fraction, intraprocedural complications, and the utilization of multiple stents.[10] In the present study, all three SES patients with SAT and six out of eight patients in the PES group had more than two drug-eluting stents implanted. There were no statistically significant differences between the two groups regarding ejection fraction and angiographic complications such as persistent slow flow, perforations, and dissections.

Antiplatelet therapy

The role of antiplatelet therapy in the prevention of SAT has been established as of great importance.[8,10,14] The Clopidogrel for the Reduction of Events During Observation (CREDO) and the PCI-CURE (PCI Clopidogrel in Unstable angina to prevent Recurrent Events) studies both indicated benefits of long-term clopidogrel therapy beyond prevention of subacute stent thrombosis.[15,16] With relative risk reductions in death and nonfatal MI to 24 and 25%, respectively, the evidence for long-term use of clopidogrel is substantial. However, clopidogrel is not universally available to all patients for economic and other (i.e. geographic) reasons. Complications after coronary-artery bypass graft (CABG) or post-noncardiac surgery in clopidogrel-treated patients are substantial; judicious use is mandated to limit potential clinical risks, particularly bleeding.[17] In our practice, we give a clopidogrel loading dose of 300 mg to those who are not pretreated.

In our study, one patient in the SES group and one patient in the PES group with SAT discontinued antiplatelet therapy before the assigned time. Another patient with LST in the SES group discontinued antiplatelet therapy (including aspirin)

10 days before the event (38 days post-stenting and before the suggested time). Recently, the possibility of drug–drug interactions with clopidogrel and statins has been scrutinized. An *ex vivo* platelet-function study suggested that the effectiveness of clopidogrel in inhibiting platelet aggregation is attenuated by co-administration of atorvastatin.[18] However, an analysis of a placebo-controlled randomized trial showed no adverse effect.[19] It is noteworthy that 82% of patients (9 out of 11 patients) who sustained SAT were on statin therapy compared with 49% of patients who did not have SAT ($p = 0.58$).

Incidence of thrombosis after SES or PES implantation

The combined (any) stent thrombosis rate at a mean follow-up of 9 months for the SES group and 7 months for the PES group was 1.47%. Overall, the incidence of AT, SAT, LST and any stent thrombosis at follow-up did not differ significantly between the two groups. The SAT rate for SES was similar to that reported in the literature ($<0.5\%$).[3,5,6] Moreover, the combined SAT rate with both SES and PES usage was 0.6%. It must also be noted that with the utilization of DES, the scope of PCI has been expanded from the more conventional indications to more aggressive types of treatment including high-risk baseline patient (i.e. diabetes, multivessel disease, poor left ventricular function) and lesion characteristics (B2 and C type lesions, total occlusions, RVD smaller than 2.5 mm, long lesions and the combination of small vessels and long lesions). In our study, more than 85% of the patient population had multivessel disease and approximately 25% were diabetics; 32% of stents had a nominal diameter smaller than 2.5 mm, with an average stent length for this size of 22.74 ± 11.63 mm.

Differences in stent thrombosis incidence between the two stent types

In the present study, we did not find any differences regarding the incidence of stent thrombosis between the two stent types. It must be noted, however, that our study was underpowered to detect any significant difference in the incidence of thrombotic events between the two stents. More specifically, a sample size of 9450 is required to achieve 80% power to detect a difference of 0.6% using a two-sided Chi-square test with continuity correction and with a significance level of 0.05. In addition, despite having similar demographics, the two groups differed in pre- and post-intervention QCA data: PES patients had a higher frequency of pre-intervention TIMI-3 flow and a shorter lesion length and larger post-procedure dimensions (but similar diameter stenosis) compared with SES patients, reflecting the nonavailability of SES larger than 3.0 mm for a time period. The question of differences (if any) in thrombogenicity between the two drug-eluting stents needs to be adressed in the ongoing and future randomized trials.

Timing and outcome of the SAT

Similary to previous reports with bare-metal stents, the majority (83%) of the SAT cases in our study occurred within 1 week post-procedure.[20,21] In our series, out of the 11 cases with SAT, 8 presented as acute MI and 3 patients died. In accordance with previously reported data, the clinical consequences of SAT were dire.[8,13,21] At the 3-month clinical follow-up, four of the eight patients (50%) with SAT presented as acute MI and suffered a major cardiac event. More specifically, two patients died, one patient underwent failed PCI which was followed by CABG, and one patient suffered recurrence of SAT treated with a new PCI. These findings are consistent with the results of Hasdai *et al.*, which showed poor clinical outcomes despite prompt restoration of blood flow after stent thrombosis.[22]

Study limitations

Several potential limitations need to be addressed. First, this was a retrospective analysis. Offsetting this limitation, the data were collected prospectively by independent monitors and entered into a dedicated database; an independent core laboratory interpreted all angiographic studies. Second, it cannot be excluded that the sole clinical event adjudicated as clinical stent thrombosis (myocardial infarction or death) was in fact due to other causes. Similary, in the absence of systematic angiographic follow-up, cases of silent stent thrombosis cannot be excluded. The latter also holds true for the incidence of late stent thrombosis rates. Moreover, the mean follow-up time was longer for the SES group reflecting the earlier availability of these stents in our centers. However, 30-day follow-up was available in all patients. In addition, the mean follow-up time was 9 months for the SES group and 7 months for the PES group, a sufficient time period for the estimation of late stent thrombosis rates. Finally, the identification of stent length and complexity (B2 or C type) of the lesion as predictors of DES thrombosis does not preclude a possible important role of other factors that are traditionally recognized in bare-metal stent studies. For statistical purposes, we had to limit the studied parameters to the most relevant (to our knowledge) clinical and procedural factors. We must also highlight the fact that the exact pathophysiology of DES thrombosis has not yet been fully elucidated, and we had to rely on factors associated with this malady in results of earlier bare-metal stent studies.

REFERENCES

1. Schomig A, Neumann FJ, Kastrati A, et al. A randomized comparison of antiplatelet and anticoagulant therapy after the placement of coronary-artery stents. N Engl J Med 1996; 334: 1084–9
2. Moussa I, Di Mario C, Reimers B, et al. Subacute stent thrombosis in the era of intravascular ultrasound-guided coronary stenting without anticoagulation: frequency, predictors and clinical outcome. J Am Coll Cardiol 1997: 6–12

3. Stone GW, Ellis SG, Cox DA, et al. A polymer-based, paclitaxel-eluting stent in patients with coronary artery disease. N Engl J Med 2004; 350: 221–31

4. Morice MC, Serruys PW, Sousa JE, et al. A randomized comparison of a sirolimus-eluting stent with a standard stent for coronary revascularization. N Engl J Med 2002; 346: 1773–80

5. Moses JW, Leon MB, Popma JJ, et al. Sirolimus-eluting stents versus standard stents in patients with stenosis in a native coronary artery. N Engl J Med 2003; 349: 1315–23

6. FDA. Information for physicians on subacute thromboses (SAT) and hypersensitivity reactions with use of the Cordis Cypher coronary stent. Public Health Web Notification Issued 10/29/03

7. Colombo A, Orlic D, Stankovic G, et al. Preliminary observations regarding angiographic pattern of restenosis after rapamycin-eluting stent implantation. Circulation 2003; 107: 2178–80

8. Cutlip DE, Baim DS, Ho KK, et al. Stent thrombosis in the modern era: a pooled analysis of multicenter coronary stent clinical trials. Circulation 2001; 103: 1967–71

9. Honda Y, Fitzgerald PJ. Stent thrombosis: an issue revisited in a changing world. Circulation 2003; 108: 2–5

10. Moussa I, Di Mario C, Reimers B, et al. Subacute stent thrombosis in the era of intravascular ultrasound-guided coronary stenting without anticoagulation: frequency, predictors and clinical outcome. J Am Coll Cardiol 1997; 29: 6–12

11. Farb A, Burke AP, Kolodgie FD, Virmani R. Pathological mechanisms of fatal late coronary stent thrombosis in humans. Circulation 2003; 108: 1701–6

12. Schuhlen H, Kastrati A, Dirschinger J, et al. Intracoronary stenting and risk for major adverse cardiac events during the first month. Circulation 1998; 98: 104–11

13. Silva JA, Ramee SR, White CJ, et al. Primary stenting in acute myocardial infarction: influence of diabetes mellitus in angiographic results and clinical outcome. Am Heart J 1999; 138: 446–55

14. Cheneau E, Leborgne L, Mintz GS, et al. Predictors of subacute stent thrombosis: results of a systematic intravascular ultrasound study. Circulation 2003; 108: 43–7

15. Steinhubl SR, Berger PB, Mann JT 3rd, et al. Early and sustained dual oral antiplatelet therapy following percutaneous coronary intervention: a randomized controlled trial. JAMA 2002; 288: 2411–20

16. Mehta SR, Yusuf S, Peters RJ, et al. Effects of pretreatment with clopidogrel and aspirin followed by long-term therapy in patients undergoing percutaneous coronary intervention: the PCI-CURE study. Lancet 2001; 358: 527–33

17. Merritt JC, Bhatt DL. The efficacy and safety of perioperative antiplatelet therapy. J Thromb Thrombolysis 2002; 13: 97–103

18. Lau WC, Waskell LA, Watkins PB, et al. Atorvastatin reduces the ability of clopidogrel to inhibit platelet aggregation: a new drug–drug interaction. Circulation 2003; 107: 32–7

19. Saw J, Steinhubl SR, Berger PB, et al. Lack of adverse clopidogrel–atorvastatin clinical interaction from secondary analysis of a randomized, placebo-controlled clopidogrel trial. Circulation 2003; 108: 921–4

20. Fischman DL, Leon MB, Baim DS, et al. A randomized comparison of coronary-stent placement and balloon angioplasty in the treatment of coronary artery disease. Stent Restenosis Study Investigators. N Engl J Med 1994; 331: 496–501

21. Serruys PW, Strauss BH, Beatt KJ, et al. Angiographic follow-up after placement of a self-expanding coronary-artery stent. N Engl J Med 1991; 324: 13–7

22. Hasdai D, Garratt KN, Holmes DR Jr., et al. Coronary angioplasty and intracoronary thrombolysis are of limited efficacy in resolving early intracoronary stent thrombosis. J Am Coll Cardiol 1996; 28: 361–7

Drug-eluting stent failures

1. Mode of failure with DES: gap and maldistribution of stent struts

Case # 11165/02

Case # 11165/02 is illustrated by **slides 1–8** (*frames 1–13* and *runs 1–4*). *Frames 1* and *2* illustrate the baseline angiogram and the result following implantation of several Cypher stents (Cordis) in order to treat a total occlusion of a right coronary artery. The occlusion of the right coronary artery represents in-stent restenosis following bare-metal stent implantation. *Frame 2* demonstrates the optimal result following implantation of Cypher stents. As indicated by the yellow arrow, there is a segment in the distal right coronary artery where there are no stents. The final result is demonstrated in *frame 3*. The 5-month follow-up is revealing because it shows a possible mode of failure of drug-eluting stents. If we examine the IVUS evaluation as shown in *frame 5* and *run 1*, we see that inside the most distal Cypher there is a minimal proliferation, and this confirms the pleasing angiographic result. When we go to the restenosis site, it is evident that there are no stent struts at that level, and the presence of restenosis is fairly obvious as demonstrated in *frame 6* and IVUS *run 2*. In the other segment, where there is focal and diffuse restenosis as shown in *frame 7* and *run 3*, a careful examination of this IVUS run shows that there are several spots of under-expanded stents with struts grossly maldistributed. This situation is certainly prone to allow proliferation in some areas where struts are not present and the drug is not delivered. The areas of narrowing near segments of stent under-expansion are evident, and most probably calcium and fibrosis contributed to this problem – a situation difficult to correct unless the lesion is well prepared at the baseline. The same issue is demonstrated in *run 4* and *frame 8*.

Message   This case exemplifies the different ways in which a drug-eluting stent may fail: no stent as in the distal right coronary artery (gap) or stent strut maldistribution owing to calcium fibrosis and stent under-expansion. Lesion preparation more than post-dilatation may become important in selected lesions to avoid this problem.

2. Another failure mode for DES: stent under-expansion

Case # 10885/02

Case # 10885/02 is illustrated by **slides 1–5** (*frames 1–12*). This is an example of distal stenosis inside a bare-metal stent treated with a Cypher stent implanted in the distal segment of a right coronary artery as demonstrated in *frame 2*. The follow-up angiogram at 9 months shows a focal restenosis inside the Cypher stent as demonstrated in *frame 3*. The IVUS evaluation at the time of follow-up (*frames 6*) and *7* shows that, in addition to tissue proliferation inside the stent, there is stent underexpansion (particularly in *frame 6*). The stent that is better expanded is the old stent, which is clearly seen as double-strut images in most of the frames. The distance between the two struts is more evident in *frame 9*, where the old stent cross-sectional area is almost identical to the vessel cross-sectional area of 16.9 mm², while the Cypher stent cross-sectional area is only 5.6 mm².

Message   In our view, this fact may explain some of the problems of focal in-stent restenosis or even diffuse disease owing to the impossibility of the drug reaching the target site in the more inner aspect of the vessel. *Frame 12* shows the final result following plain balloon angioplasty with a high-pressure balloon.

3. Stent under-expansion and strut maldistribution as possible causes for restenosis in DES

Case MEN/HSR

Case MEN/HSR is illustrated by **slides 1–3** (*frames 1–7*). The baseline lesion is in the distal part of the right coronary artery as demonstrated in *frame 1* and was treated successfully with a long 3-mm Cypher stent as demonstrated in *frame 2*. The final result is demonstrated in *frame 3*, with the follow-up angiogram showing a focal restenosis inside the Cypher stent. A careful examination of *frame 3* demonstrates that in the area where restenosis occurred, the result was not optimal as in the other segment of the Cypher stent. The IVUS evaluation is shown in *frame 5*. It is obvious from *frame 7* that in the area of restenosis the stent is under-expanded, the struts are unevenly distributed, and there is calcium and fibrosis.

Message   Again, this case reiterates what we have already said regarding the contribution of poor lesion preparation and poor stent expansion to the development of restenosis following drug-eluting stent implantation.

4. Severe stent under-expansion: a possible cause of DES restenosis

Case # 10738/02

This is a case of diffuse multifocal in-stent restenosis following Cypher stent implantation in a patient with diabetes and unstable angina (**slides 1–3** (*frames 1–9*)). The lesion involves an occlusion of the distal right coronary artery and a stenosis at the ostium of an acute marginal branch. Both these vessels were stented with multiple

Cypher stents. The final result of the original procedure is shown in *frame 2*, and the 6-month follow-up is shown in *frame 3*. There is multifocal restenosis in the distal right and a focal stenosis in the proximal acute marginal branch. IVUS evaluation performed in the distal right coronary artery shows gross stent under-expansion immediately distal to the bifurcation, with a combination of hyperplasia and stent under-expansion. Note the fibro-calcific plaque behind the stent. In the more distal part, the stent is better expanded with a more symmetrical appearance and no hyperplasia. This restenosis was treated with simple angioplasty, and the 6-month follow-up shows a sustained patency for both branches.

Message   We still do not know the best approach to treat Cypher restenosis. IVUS evaluation should probably be part of this procedure.

5. Is stent under-expansion a real cause of in-stent restenosis?

Case # 10994/02

This case (**slides 1** and **2** (*frames 1–11*)) illustrates an evaluation of in-stent restenosis after 11 months of Cypher stent implantation in the left anterior descending in various segments. The most proximal lesion, visible in *frame 1*, is an in-stent restenosis of the first stent which, evaluated by IVUS in *frame 2*, is under-expanded. *Frames 4* and *5* show again the same findings with hyperplasia and gross stent under-expansion compared with the size of the vessel. In the same vessel, we see other areas of stent under-expansion, as demonstrated in *frames 7–11*, in which a stent under-expansion was not associated with hyperplasia or restenosis. It is not clear why in some circumstances stent under-expansion is associated with hyperplasia but in other circumstances it is not. Of course, in biology not every event is repeatable 100% of the time, and even if stent under-expansion may cause drug maldistribution and hyperplasia, this fact does not mean that the correlation always has to be 1:1.

Message   Despite our belief that stent under-expansion may be an important element that leads to in-stent restenosis, there is not yet a convincing demonstration.

6. Gaps, strut maldistribution, and stent under-expansion: possible causes for restenosis in a DES

Case # 11127/02

This case (**slides 1–6** (*frames 1–20*)) illustrates, in a single patient, multiple modes of drug-eluting stent failure as a possible cause of in-stent restenosis or peri-stent restenosis. The baseline angiogram shows a long lesion with a bifurcational lesion in the circumflex and obtuse marginal branch (*frame 1*). The procedure was successfully completed following implantation of multiple Cypher stents, including full coverage of the bifurcational lesion using the crush technique without final kissing. At follow-up (*frame 4*), we see multifocal restenosis in the main circumflex at the ostium of the obtuse marginal branch and in the body of the stent of the obtuse marginal branch.

IVUS interrogation gave us multiple insights into the possible mechanisms of restenosis. The first finding is in *frame 8*, and the IVUS (*frame 5*) shows that the restenotic site is not covered by any stent strut (gap). We can say that stent gaps are a possible cause of restenosis. The next finding is seen in *frame 12* and the IVUS (*frame 9*): we notice that compared with *frame 10*, the distance from the stent struts to the internal elastic lamina is almost three to four times. This stent under-expansion may affect the delivery of the drug to the target site. The other mechanism is seen in *frame 16* and the IVUS image in *frame 13*. In the IVUS (*frame 13*), we notice mal-distribution of the stent struts associated with under-expansion. Maldistribution of stent struts can be a cause of inhomogeneous drug delivery and can affect the ability of the drug to limit hyperplasia. The last example, which is similar to the previous one, is more clearly illustrated in the IVUS (*frame 17*), where (based on the clock face) all the struts are together at 12 o'clock and no other strut is visible in the other part of the vessel where there is maximum hyperplasia, for example at 6 o'clock.

Message   We believe that some of the above mechanisms are certainly implicated in causing in-stent restenosis. Again, careful vessel preparation and optimization of stent delivery with IVUS guidance can avoid some of these problems. We do not advocate this type of strategy on approaching every lesion, but when dealing with diffuse disease and long lesions, an approach with IVUS guidance and careful lesion preparation may be important.

7. A constant 'traction' at a site of implantation of a DES as a possible cause of excess proliferation

Case # 10297/01

This case is illustrated by **slides 1–4** (*frames 1–11*). The patient presented with a long lesion at the obtuse marginal branch of the circumflex following failure of a saphenous vein graft anastomosed to that vessel.

The lesion was treated with elective implantation of two Cypher stents as demonstrated in *frames 2* and *3* with the final result shown in *frame 5*. The follow-up angiogram, triggered by symptoms shown in *frame 6*, demonstrates a focal restenosis in the distal part of the stent. This area is clearly inside the stent as demonstrated by careful examination of the angiogram. The patient underwent implantation of another Cypher stent as demonstrated in *frame 8* with an optimal final result as shown in *frame 9*. Following a few months, the patient again became symptomatic, and a second restenosis is seen at the site of the first restenosis – almost a carbon copy of the first failure. Careful examination of this angiogram shows traction exerted by the graft at the site of the anastomosis; possibly these extra forces gave an additional stress to the area affecting the shear forces distribution and contributing to the increased proliferation. Owing to the multiple failures, we decided to implant two Cypher stents together, one inside the other, utilizing the sandwich technique. The final result following this procedure is shown in *frame 11*. So far, following more than the 1-year follow-up, the patient remains asymptomatic, and it is very likely that this final procedure was successful.

Message   Abnormal shear stress can be an additional cause of restenosis in a DES.

8. A transient 'restenosis'

Case JM

This case is illustrated by **slides 1–4** (*frames 1–8*). *Frames 1* and *2* show an image with which we were familiar in the past when utilizing radioactive stents. This image, particularly the one in the postero-lateral branch (*frame 1*) is a typical candy-wrapper appearance. Initially, the impression was a proximal and distal peri-stent restenosis. The surprise came following nitroglycerin administration with complete disappearance of the above lesions as illustrated in *frames 3* and *4*. This fact gives more emphasis to the usual strategy to administer nitroglycerin during each angiogram, a strategy sometimes forgotten and of paramount importance in order not only to evaluate the presence of a true lesion but also to give the operator a quick impression of the true size of the vessel to be treated.

Message   An angiogram is not diagnostic unless taken after intracoronary nitroglycerin administration.

8

A View from the USA

Experience with drug-eluting stents

Giora Weisz MD, *Jeffrey W Moses* MD

Case 1 – Diffuse LAD disease

History

Case 1 is illustrated by **slides 1** and **2** (*frames 1–4*). A 72-year-old man with type-II diabetes mellitus and hypercholesterolemia was referred for coronary intervention due to severe angina (Canadian Cardiovascular Society stage III), despite maximal anti-anginal therapy.

Diagnostic angiography

Angiography showed normal left ventricular function. The right coronary artery and the left circumflex (LCX) had diffuse nonobstructive disease. The left anterior descending artery (LAD) had diffuse calcified disease with stenosis up to 90% in its proximal and mid segments (*frame 1*). A bifurcating diagonal branch is taking-off at the mid-LAD lesion.

Intervention

The planned strategy was to wire the diagonal branch in addition to the LAD, in order to preserve side-branch access. An 8-Fr guide-catheter XB 3.5 (Cordis) with side holes was introduced into the left main coronary artery. This size of guide was selected in order to provide good support while stenting long diffuse disease and to enable delivery and deployment of two stents at the bifurcation. Using a Balance Universal (Guidant) guide-wire, it was unable to access the diagonal branch, so only the LAD was wired. A pre-dilatation of the mid and proximal LAD with a 3.0×15-mm balloon (Fx Minirail, Guidant) was carried out in order to prepare the vessel for stent deployment. Pre-dilatation of long diffuse calcified artery helped achieve smoother deliverability of the stent. Furthermore, pre-dilatation of calcified vessel will make the artery more concentric (round) so the drug will elute from the stent to the vessel uniformly. The balloon dilatation across the diagonal branch (*frame 2*), made a conformational change with possible plaque shift that 'helped' to provide access to the branch and to wire it (*frame 3*). Two Cypher stents were deployed. First, in the mid LAD, a 3.0×28-mm stent, and a second proximal overlapping 3.5×33-mm stent that extends to the ostial LAD. The final angiogram revealed good angiograpic results without affecting the ostial LCX (*frame 4*).

Case 2 – Tortuous RCA

History

Case 2 is illustrated by slides 1–5 (*frames 1–10*). A 67-year-old man with hyper-tension, type-II diabetes mellitus and hypercholesterolemia was referred for coronary intervention due to severe angina (Canadian Cardiovascular Society stage III), despite maximal anti-anginal therapy. The patient had prior interventions of his left anterior descending artery and left circumflex/obtuse marginal bifurcation, and had mildly reduced left ventricular function.

Diagnostic angiography

The right coronary artery was a very tortuous route with an anomalous anterior take-off (*frames 1, 2*).

Intervention

The challenges in this case included good guide-catheter support in a very tortuous artery with anomalous origin, negotiating a guide-wire through the loops and lesions, and delivering long drug-eluting stents through the tortuous vessel. A 6-Fr Ampltaz 1.0 guide-catheter was chosen for artery cannulation. A 0.014″ Dasher wire (Boston Scientific) with a high degree of torque was chosen first, but was not able to be advanced beyond the second loop (*frames 3–5*). Additional wires, including a Pilot 50 wire (Guidant), Balance Universal, and PT2 moderate-support (Boston Scientific) were also unable to be advanced further down the artery. During these attempts, there was suboptimal support from the guide-catheter, so it was replaced with a 7-Fr multipurpose guide-catheter with side holes, which could be engaged more deeply and provide better support (*frame 6*).

The hydrophilic Pilot 50 wire was used again through a transit catheter which provided sub-selective support through the loops of the tortuous artery. This strategy was successful, and wire was advanced distally (*frame 7*). Note the wire bias seen because of straightening of the vessel. In this situation, the operator needs full understanding of lesion locations, with help of markers such as side branches. The two lesions were pre-dilated with 2.5×15-mm balloon (Maverick 2). A 2.5×20-mm

Taxus stent was successfully advanced and deployed at the distal lesion segment (*frame 8*). Two additional Cypher stents were deployed proximally, to cover the long diffuse disease, with a good final result (*frames 9, 10*).

Case 3 – Multi-vessel and bifurcation stenting

History

Case 3 is illustrated by slides 1–6 (*frames 1–11*). A 74-year-old man was referred for coronary angiography because of stable angina pectoris that was not improved with medical therapy. He had a prior stent placement in the right coronary artery (RCA).

Diagnostic angiography

Coronary angiography revealed a patent stent in the RCA. The left anterior descending artery (LAD) had a bifurcational lesion, 90% stenosis of the mid LAD with involvement of the ostial diagonal branch (*frame 1*). The proximal left circumflex artery (LCX) had an 80% stenosis (*frame 2*). Left ventricular function was normal.

Intervention

An 8-Fr EBU guide-catheter (Medtronic) was used to allow simultaneous deployment of two stents using the 'crush' technique. First, the LCX was treated. The strategy of direct stenting was chosen since the artery was not calcified and not tortuous, and the lesion was not tight. A 3.5×23-mm Cypher stent was successfully deployed, with an appearance of proximal edge dissection (*frame 3*). Another Cypher stent 3.5×8-mm was deployed, minimally overlapping the first stent and covering the dissection (*frame 4*).

The LAD-diagonal bifurcation was treated using the 'crush' technique. This technique is based on simultaneous positioning of two stents in the two branches, in such a way that the side-branch stent is protruding into the main branch, to verify complete coverage of the angled ostium of the branch. The principle of complete coverage of the side-branch ostium is particularly important with the use of drug-eluting stents. Thus, full coverage of all parts of the bifurcation with anti-proliferative medication is achieved. Some tips described below enable safe and successful 'crushing'. First, it is useful to use different lengths of wires to ease discrimination between the two during all parts of the procedure. In the current case, a 300-cm BMW Universal wire (Guidant) was introduced into the LAD, and a similar 190-cm wire into the diagonal branch. Second, a good preparation of the vessels, i.e. pre-dilatation is important. This can be done by a kissing balloon inflation, here with two 2.5×15-mm Maverick balloons (*frame 5*), and demonstrating that there is a good lumen for successful stent delivery (*frame 6*).

Before deploying the stents, the operator and his assistant should certainly be sure as to which stent goes to which artery. The different lengths of the wires help to differentiate between the target branches. Our routine is to prepare (negative aspiration) only the side-branch stent. The main-vessel stent is positioned without preparation, and without connection to an end-deflator. This precaution will prevent first deployment of the main-vessel stent. Once this occurs, the delivery balloon of the side branch may be locked, and the operator might be unable to pull it out. Thus, after careful positioning of both stents, the side-branch stent is deployed first (Cypher stent, 2.5×18 mm, *frame 7*). The delivery balloon and wire are pulled from the side branch, to prevent their lock by the second stent. Then, the second (main-vessel) stent is deployed (Cypher stent, 3.0×33 mm, *frame 8*), 'crushing' the proximal protruding portion of the first stent aside, to the vessel wall.

The next step is post-dilatation of both stents. The side branch is re-crossed (in our experience, successful in 90% of cases). Post-dilatation balloons (here two 2.5×15-mm Maverick balloons, *frame 9*) are positioned *inside* the stent margins and inflated (and deflated) simultaneously, to ensure maximal apposition of the stent struts at the bifurcation. In some cases, the balloon does not cross the side branch. This problem can be usually solved by initial dilatation with a 1.5-mm balloon. The final result is excellent (*frames 10, 11*).

Case 4 – Stent ablation

History

Case 4 is illustrated by **slides 1–4** (*frames 1–8*). Two months before the current procedure, in another institution, a 42-year-old man had a 3.0×28-mm Cypher stent deployed in his right coronary artery (RCA). Pre-dilatation in this calcified artery was not performed, and the operators were unable to dilate fully the stent. The patient was referred for further evaluation and treatment because of continued exertional angina.

Diagnostic angiography and intervention

Using a 9-Fr JR4 guide-catheter with side-holes, an angiogram of the RCA showed severe stenosis in the middle of the stent (*frame 1*). A BMW Universal wire crossed the lesion, but an IVUS-guided catheter as well as a Maverick 1.5×9-mm balloon were unable to cross the lesion. The plan at this point was to try to 'ablate' the stent with a rotational atherectomy device (Rotablator, Boston Scientific), to allow balloon expansion of the old stent, and placement of a new drug-eluting stent. Rotational ablation, even of metal, is expected to produce microparticles that are too small to damage the heart, and are taken up in the lungs and the reticuloendothelial system. After changing to a Rotablator extra-support wire, a 1.25-mm Rotablator burr (*frame 2*) was advanced, followed by a 1.5-mm burr, but despite repeated attempts, both were unable to cross the lesion. Another attempt to cross the lesion with the 1.5-mm balloon failed, even after changing to a stiff wire (Ironman). Since the guide-catheter was not providing sufficient support, it was changed to an 8-Fr AL 0.75 (an AL 1.0 guide did not fit) (*frame 3*). Even after repeat trials with the Rotablator 1.5-mm burr, the 1.5-mm balloon did not cross the lesion.

Using the Spectranetics sub-sheath catheter (its end-hole wedged at the lesion) the Rota wire was exchanged for a 0.014″ BMW Universal wire, and later to a Wiggle wire (Guidant). The idea for using the Wiggle wire was that the struts of the stent could possibly prevent further advancement of the balloon. The Wiggle wire may divert the balloon tip to allow passage. This strategy was found to be helpful in this case. The operator was able to cross the lesion with the 1.5-mm balloon and inflate it up to 22 atm. A larger balloon could not cross. A Pivot 2.5-mm balloon was successfully used (*frame 4*). This balloon is not delivered on a wire, but rather has a short wire at its tip, thus allowing a low profile and the ability to be pushed. Even after dilatation with the Pivot balloon, another 2.5-mm over-the-wire low-profile balloon (Maverick) could not cross. The Rotablator system was re-introduced. Surprisingly, although the 1.25-mm burr passage was not successful, the 1.5-mm burr was able to pass through the lesion, by ablating the metal. It was followed by a 1.75-mm burr to increase further the lumen (*frame 5*).

After the 'stent ablation' the lesion could be crossed by 2.5×15-mm Crossail balloon (Guidant), followed by noncompliant balloons in increasing size: 3.0×15-mm Powersail, 3.5×15-mm Powersail, and Quantum 3.75×15-mm (which ruptured at 18 atm), and 4.0×15-mm Powersail, leading to increased lumen size (*frame 6*). A long segment of the RCA was stented with three Cypher stents, 23 mm + 23 mm + 18 mm, overlapping each other and covering all segments of injury. Stents of 3.0 mm in diameter were used (larger stents were not available), and post-dilated with a 4.0-mm balloon (Crossail), with an excellent angiographic result (*frames 7, 8*).

Case 5 – Acute myocardial infarction

History

Case 5 is illustrated by **slides 1–7** (*frames 1–13*). A 45-year-old man without prior medical history was admitted 2 h after the beginning of severe sub-sternal chest pain and was hemodynamically stable; ECG revealed ST segment elevation on the precordial leads. The patient received oral aspirin (325 mg), clopidogrel (600 mg), and sub-lingual nitroglycerin, and was started on intra-venous heparin.

Diagnostic angiography

A coronary angiogram showed thrombotic occlusion of the left anterior descending artery (LAD) at the bifurcation with a diagonal branch (*frame 1*). The right coronary artery had minimal luminal irregularities. The left ventriculogram showed reduced left ventricle (LV) function with anterior hypokinesis.

Intervention

An 8-Fr VL 3.5 guide-catheter was chosen to enable simultaneous negotiation and treatment of the main artery and the side branch. A temporary pacemaker wire was inserted through the femoral vein and placed in the right ventricle for back-up. Immediately after inserting wires (BMW Universal) into the LAD and the diagonal branch, reconstitution of flow was demonstrated (*frame 2*), but a large thrombus mass remained in the diagonal branch. An Angiojet catheter (Possis) was advanced first into the LAD, and later into the diagonal (*frame 3*). Two passes were made in each vessel, without significant improvement (*frame 4*). The bifurcation segment was dilated with a 2.5 × 15-mm Maverick balloon in both the LAD and the diagonal, without improvement in the tight stenosis in the ostial diagonal branch and with continued slow flow in both branches.

Because of the large thrombus mass in the diagonal branch, a Filterwire EZ (Boston Scientific) distal protection device was introduced to the distal diagonal branch, to prevent distal embolization (*frame 5*). The ostial diagonal was dilated with a 3.0 × 10-mm cutting balloon (Boston Scientific), so a 3.0 × 33-mm Cypher stent was introduced and deployed in the mid portion of the diagonal branch (*frame 6*). The distal protection filter was removed, followed by stenting of the bifurcation, using the 'crush technique'. A 3.0 × 18-mm Cypher stent in the diagonal branch and a 3.5 × 18-mm Cypher stent in the LAD were positioned. First, the side-branch (diagonal) stent was deployed (*frame 7*), followed by withdrawal of its delivery balloon and wire, and then deployment of the LAD stent (*frame 8*). A repeat angiogram showed wide dilatation of the LAD, with a suboptimal result at the diagonal ostium (*frame 9*). After rewiring of the diagonal branch, a kissing balloon dilatation was performed using a 3.0 × 15-mm Quantum balloon (Boston Scientific) in the diagonal, and a 3.5 × 15-mm Quantum balloon in the LAD (*frame 10*), with good final angiographic results (*frame 11*) and flow.

Case 6 – PCI of native coronary arteries in patient with prior CABG

History

Case 6 is illustrated by slides 1–4 (*frames 1–7*). A 68-year-old man with hypertension, type-II diabetes mellitus, hypercholesterolemia and prior (10 year) CABG surgery (LIMA to LAD, SVG to OM). He was referred for coronary intervention due to severe angina (Canadian Cardiovascular Society stage III), despite maximal antianginal therapy. A nuclear stress-test demonstrated a fixed perfusion defect at the inferior wall, and reversible perfusion defects at the anterior, anterior-lateral, apical, and inferior-apical walls.

Diagnostic angiography

The ostial left anterior descending artery (LAD) had a significant stenosis involving the distal left main coronary artery (LMCA), and was occluded immediately after take-off of a large diagonal branch that had a long diffuse stenosis (*frames 1, 2*). The left circumflex artery was occluded at its proximal part. The right coronary artery was occluded. The saphenous vein graft to the obtuse marginal branch (OM) was also found to be occluded. The LIMA to distal LAD was patent with moderate tortuosity (*frame 3*), patent anastomosis, but an 80% stenosis in the LAD distal to the anastomosis (*frame 4*). The LAD also supplies collaterals to the posterior descending branch of the RCA. Left ventricular systolic function was reduced with an ejection fraction of 35%, and a +1 mitral regurgitation.

Intervention

The planned strategy in this case was revascularization of the ischemic myocardial areas by dilatation and stenting of the native LAD and diagonal branch.

A 6-Fr EBU 3.5 guide-catheter (Medtronic) was used to engage the native left coronary system. The proximal LAD–diagonal branch was crossed with a BMW wire. Pre-dilatation was performed with a 2.5×20-mm Maverick balloon. Partial dilatation of the long-standing calcified artery was achieved and smooth delivery of the long stent was allowed. In addition, pre-dilatation leads to a more circular final geometry of the artery, so there will be equal distances between stent struts and uniform distribution of the sirolimus to the vessel wall. A 3.0×13-mm Cypher stent covered the distal LMCA/ostial LAD (*frames 5, 6*).

For the distal LAD intervention, a short (90 cm) 6-Fr IMA guide-catheter was taken to engage the LIMA through the subclavian artery. The same wire was used to cross the native distal LAD through the LIMA. The lesion was pre-dilated with a 2.5×20-mm Maverick balloon. The 2.5×18-mm Cypher stent was easily delivered through the LIMA tortuosity and deployed (*frame 7*)

Case 7 – Distal LMCA

History

Case 7 is illustrated by **slides 1–8** (*frames 1–16*). A 55-year-old man with hypertension and hypercholesterolemia was admitted due to new-onset angina on minimal exertion.

Diagnostic angiography

The proximal left coronary system was calcified. The distal left main coronary artery (LMCA) had a 90% stenosis that extended into the ostial left anterior descending artery (LAD) and involved also the ostial circumflex artery (LCX). The proximal LCX had a 80% focal stenosis, and the obtuse marginal branch (OM) had a focal moderate stenosis (*frame 1*). The right coronary artery had nonobstructive irregularities.

Revascularization options were discussed with the patient, who refused surgical procedure and elected for percutaneous intervention.

Intervention

During LMCA intervention, it is important to monitor meticulously all hemo-dynamic parameters, and to be able to cope with any possible deterioration. An intra-aortic balloon pump was inserted for hemodynamic support during the intervention.

An 8-Fr XB 3 guide-catheter (Cordis) was used to engage the native left coro-nary system (an XB 3.5 did not fit). The LAD and LCX were wired with a BMW Universal wire. Because of the significant calcification of the lesion, a 3.5×6-mm cutting balloon (Boston Scientific) was chosen. Delivered over the LCX wire, and positioned across the distal LMCA into the LCX (*frame 2*), several very short infla-tions of the cutting balloon partially relieved the tight stenosis (*frame 3*). IVUS interrogation showed that both arteries had a reference diameter of 3.5 mm, still with a stenosis of 80–90%, and that the focal stenosis of the OM was significant (90%). The LCX and OM lesions were dilated with a 3.0×6-mm cutting balloon (*frame 4*). A 3.0×23-mm Cypher stent was deployed successfully in the OM branch (*frame 5*). The distal LMCA bifurcation was stented using the 'crush' technique. A Cypher stent (3.5×28 mm) was positioned in the LAD and LCX in such a way that the proximal edge of the LCX extended a little into the LMCA to cover fully the LCX ostium (*frame 6*). The LCX stent was deployed first (*frame 7*), and, after pulling out the delivery balloon and wire, the LAD stent was deployed as well (*frame 8*).

Despite a good angiographic appearance (*frame 9*), post-dilatation is always recommended, to ensure maximal apposition of the stents to the vessel wall. The LCX was rewired, and a 1.5×15-mm Maverick balloon was inflated at the ostial LCX, in order to dilate the opening between the struts of the LAD stent that 'jail' the origin of the LCX (*frame 10*). This enabled the delivery and dilatation of a balloon that has a larger crossing profile – a 3.5×15-mm Quantum balloon (*frame 11*). Using another identical balloon, a brief kissing balloon inflation was carried out (*frame 12*). Angiography showed well-dilated LMCA and proximal segments of the LAD and LCX (*frame 13*). The gap between the two LCX stents was stented with a 3.0×13-mm Cypher stent, with excellent angiographic results (*frames 14, 15*). Repeat IVUS interrogation confirmed full apposition of the stents. The measured cross-sectional area of the LMCA was 14 mm² and of the proximal LAD 8.5 mm². The patient became asymptomatic and had a follow-up angiography 6 months later. The LMCA, LAD, and LCX were widely patent (*frame 16*). Left ventricular function was normal.

Case 8 – Thrombotic SVG

History

Case 8 is illustrated by **slides 1–7** (*frames 1–14*). An 80-year-old man with hypertension, diabetes mellitus, and hypercholesterolemia was admitted because of non-Q-wave myocardial infarction manifested by transient rest angina and elevated troponin levels. He had experienced anterior-wall MI and CABG surgery 10 years earlier, and then congestive heart failure, and had been fitted with a permanent pacemaker. At admission, the patient was pain-free and stable hemodynamically.

Diagnostic angiography

Coronary angiography performed the next day showed occluded proximal LAD, occluded LCX after a patent OM1, and patent RCA. The LIMA to mid LAD was patent with mild distal LAD disease. The SVG to D1 was patent. The saphenous vein graft (SVG) to distal OM branch had a thrombotic occlusion (*frame 1*). Intravenous integrillin infusions were started.

Intervention

A long (45 cm) sheath (Arrow) was needed because of tortuosity of the iliac artery. A 7-Fr hockey-stick type guide-catheter with side-holes was used. The plan was to use a distal protection device to protect from distal embolization of thrombotic material. The SVG was wired with a Pilot 50 wire over an Ultrafuse X catheter (Boston Scientific), but repeat injections of contrast did not demonstrate the distal segment of the SVG and the distal native artery (*frame 2*). The Ultrafuse X catheter was advanced over the wire, and injection was administered to try to determine whether the distal segment is appropriate for placement of the protection device. The distal segment was not opacified, probably because of the existence of extensive thrombus (*frame 3*).

   After exchanging different wires including Balance Universal, Dashe, and Prowater wire (Asahi Intec, Japan), the operator was able to advance further the last wire into the proximal arm of the native OM artery (*frame 4*). In order to advance a thrombectomy device, low-pressure (4 atm) pre-dilatation was carried out with a 2.0×15-mm Maverick balloon (*frame 5*). This was followed by use of rheolitic thrombectomy by the Angiojet XVG 5F (Possis) (*frame 6*). The Angiojet successfully removed the thrombus from the proximal segment of the vein, but because of the right angle at the anastomosis, it was unable to extract the distal thrombus. Thrombotic material from the distal segment was aspirated using the export catheter of the PercuSurge Guardwire system (Medtronic), with partial improvement (*frame 7*). A Balance Universal wire was directed into the distal OM, and the narrowed anastomosis was dilated with the 2.0×15-mm balloon, with improved distal flow (*frame 8*). The aspiration catheter was used again to aspirate a mobile thrombus that remained in the distal segment of the vein. A 3.5×23-mm Cypher stent was deployed at the distal segment of the SVG, proximal to the anastomosis (*frame 9*). Another 2.5×18-mm Cypher stent was deployed at the anastomosis site, minimally overlapping the first stent (*frame 10*). The proximal part of the OM was lost. The Distal edge dissection was covered with a 2.5×8-mm stent, with good final angiographic result (*frame 11*), and flow.

9

Noninvasive Evaluation

Stress echo in percutaneous coronary interventions – should anything be changed in the drug-eluting stent era?

Miodrag Ostojic MD, *Vladan Vukcevic* MD, *Eugenio Picano* MD

SUBSTANTIAL ROLE OF STRESS ECHOCARDIOGRAPHY

Coronary artery revascularization with percutaneous transluminal coronary angioplasty is an effective therapeutic procedure in the management of properly selected patients with coronary artery disease. For patient selection and assessment of procedure efficacy, a functional evaluation of stenosis is mandatory. As stated by Gruntzig at the dawn of the angioplasty era, 'imaging postcatheterization permits evaluation of the physiologic significance of an observed lesion and to determine the potential effect of dilatation on perfusion distal to the lesion'.[1] In addition, a preangioplasty imaging evaluation 'provides a baseline for noninvasive post-angioplasty monitoring of the procedure's success. As with the patient who has undergone bypass surgery, subjective symptoms are usually a good guide, but are not sufficient for the longitudinal evaluation of the procedure'.[1] The practical impact of stress echocardiography in assessing coronary angioplasty has been widely demonstrated.[2–18] The main tasks of physiological testing in angioplasty patients can be summarized as follows:

- Anatomical identification of disease and geographical localization, with physiological assessment of stenosis of intermediate anatomical severity and identification of target lesion in multivessel disease
- Risk stratification to identify asymptomatic patients more likely to benefit, in terms of survival, from a revascularization procedure
- Identification of myocardial viability in region with dyssynergy at rest
- Identification of restenosis or disease progression

It is also easy to assess the results of the revascularization procedure, which may be completely successful (with disappearance of inducible ischemia; slide 1, Figure 1) or partially successful (with persisting inducible ischemia; slide 2, Figure 2).

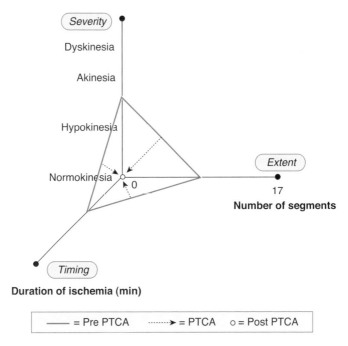

Figure 1 A completely successful percutaneous transluminal coronary angioplasty (PTCA). Following the intervention, the stress echocardiography test becomes completely negative, ideally placed at the origin of the system of coordinates localizing the stress-induced ischemia. (Modified from Picano,[21] with permission)

The timing of postangioplasty stress echocardiography varies widely, ranging from 24 h to 1 week in the various studies. All of these studies demonstrated a comparable reduction in stress echocardiography positivity rates, ranging from 70 to 100% before angioplasty and from 10 to 30% after angioplasty.[19] Stress echocardiography testing performed early after percutaneous transluminal coronary angioplasty does not seem to suffer from the reduced specificity that limits the usefulness of perfusion stress testing in this setting[20] and can be linked to the transient reduction in coronary flow reserve for reversible microvascular damage.[21] The possible physiological benefit on the regional coronary reserve determined by revascularization appears to be the most likely explanation for the improvement in stress test results. A consistently positive stress echocardiography test after angioplasty has an unfavorable prognostic implication, placing the patient in a subset at high risk for recurrence of symptoms.[8,12] The limited, or even total, lack of improvement in the test response after angiographically successful angioplasty may have several explanations. The residual stenosis may be anatomically insignificant and yet hemodynamically important because there is a poor correlation between the percentage of lumen reduction and regional flow

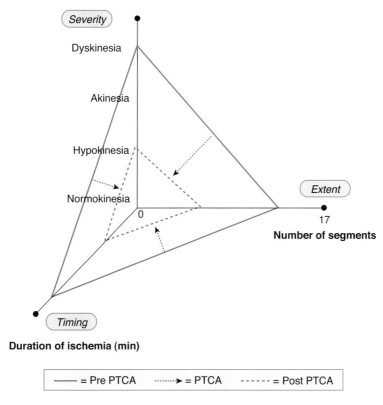

Duration of ischemia (min)

——— = Pre PTCA   ·······➤ = PTCA   – – – – – = Post PTCA

Figure 2   A partially successful percutaneous transluminal coronary angioplasty (PTCA). The severity of the ischemic response is proportional to the area of the triangle, whose vertices are placed on the coordinates of ischemia. The area obviously shrinks following intervention, but the test remains positive, suggesting a primary failure, an incomplete revascularization, or an early restenosis. (Modified from Picano,[21] with permission)

reserve, particularly very early after angioplasty. Restenosis may be difficult to recognize on postangioplasty angiograms because of the apparent improvement in luminal dimensions secondary to extravasation of contrast into the media to the plaque, with fissuring and dissection.

Among all possible imaging procedures, stress echo has obvious cost and feasibility advantages. Compared with the treadmill exercise test, the cost of stress echocardiography is at least 2.1 times higher, stress SPECT myocardial imaging 5.7 times higher, and coronary angiography 21.7 times higher.[20] In addition, stress echo has no biological burden and no radiation hazard, which is particularly important in patients submitted to angiography and angioplasty, and often more than once. A coronary angiography with stent corresponds to a dose exposure of about 1250 chest

X-rays. To this unavoidable and life-saving therapeutic exposure, it would be wise not to add the avoidable exposure of serial stress scintigraphy, each one corresponding to at least 500 chest X-rays. Radiation damage is cumulative, and a strategy of noninvasive follow-up in these patients with serial nonionizing testing is certainly highly desirable and is much more sustainable for both society and the patient.[21]

CONTEMPORARY DILEMMAS

In the stenting era, there were case reports of stent thrombosis which might be induced by stress testing.[22–25] Recently, a randomized study in 1000 post-stent patients in whom exercise stress-testing was performed within 1 day after procedure, demonstrated no increased risk of stent thrombosis (1% exercise stress group vs. 1% nonexercise stress group)[26]. Fears over performing stress-testing in patients in whom drug-eluting stents (DES) were implanted because of delayed re-endothelization therefore appear to be unjustified, as the first day after implantation bare-metal stent is totally denuded. Nevertheless, there have not been reported large-scale trials applying stress-tests in patients after DES implantation. The above-mentioned facts together with case reports of spontaneous late stent thrombosis in brachy-therapy treated patients[27] as well as in patients treated with DES[28], which can be attributed to delayed re-endothelization and/or local drug toxic effects and hypersensitivity,[29] raise concerns that any form of stress test may have adverse effects in those groups of patients.[30–34] At present, there are no clear-cut recommendations in the existing guidelines[35] for applying stress tests in patients treated with DES.

Intuitively, in the majority of hospitals, stress-testing after DES implantation is not advised before 3 months have elapsed. For the time being, there is a trade-off in each individual case between applying stress-testing to detect restenosis and/or progression of disease in nonstented vessels versus the small possibility of provoking stent thrombosis. In favor of testing is the argument that some patients, by profession, are exposed to physical efforts, so it is better if the stent thrombosis should happen to occur in a hospital where emergency PCI or thrombolysis could be performed. To demonstrate that dilemma, the following case is presented. To our knowledge, this represents one of the first cases in which late stent thrombosis occurred after exercise stress-echo testing in a patient 5 months after DES implantation. To put this data in perspective, one should consider that stress-testing (with or without associated imaging) is not a totally risk-free diagnostic procedure. The risk of major complications is about 1 in 300–500 tests for dobutamine,[36] 1 in 1000–1500 for dipyridamole,[37] and 1 in 2000–3000 for exercise.[35] In the context of stenting, it may be relevant – at least in theory – to know that some stresses (and particularly dobutamine) may have a delayed pro-aggregant effect, more obvious at 30–45 min after the end of the infusion.[38] Such an effect is independent of induced ischemia and may account for some late complications observed, more frequently with dobutamine – at the end of negative testing.[36] In addition, exercise results in activation of both the coagulation and fibrinolytic cascades, but coagulation may remain activated after fibrinolysis has returned to baseline levels.[39]

CASE REPORT

We present a case of a male patient born in 1943. The risk factors for coronary artery disease include hypercholesterolemia and smoking. His history of symptomatic coronary artery disease started in 1985 when he had his first balloon angioplasty in the proximal LAD. He was asymptomatic after that procedure, and he performed exercise stress-echo testing on a regular annual basis according to the protocol at our hospital. He was treated with 150 mg of aspirin *per os* daily and metoprolol 50 mg *per os* twice daily. He became symptomatic again in September 2002, with symptoms of effort angina. The coronary angiography, performed in September 2002 after the positive stress-echo test on stage II of Bruce protocol, revealed diffuse coronary artery disease (slide 3, Figure 3) with two significant stenoses, one in the proximal and mid portion of the LAD, and the second in the big distal circumflex. After pretreatment with ticlopidine 250 mg twice daily for 5 days, a PCI procedure was performed on 24 October 2002 with implantation of 3×33-mm Cypher stent in the proximal to mid LAD with 16 atm inflation, and balloon angioplasty with a 3.0×20-mm balloon on the circumflex with 12 atm inflation, with a good post-procedural result (slide 4, Figure 4). He was discharged on aspirin, ticlopidine, metoprolol, and atorvastatin.

According to the hospital protocol, he was scheduled for stress-echo tests at 2 and then 6 months post-procedure. The 2-month stress-echo test was negative for myocardial ischemia. Exercise was stopped at level III of Bruce protocol, at a heart rate of 126/min because of the chest pain, but without ST segment denivelation and without regional wall motion abnormalities on echo immediately after the physical effort. He was asymptomatic when he came for the 6-month stress-echo test on 26 March 2003. The test was performed at 8 o'clock in the morning, and was stopped at level II of Bruce protocol, at a heart rate of 142/min (slide 5, Figure 5). During and after the test, the patient was asymptomatic, without ECG changes or wall motion abnormalities. He was advised to continue with double antiplatelet therapy for a further 10 days, until the full 6 months following the procedure. Back at home, he started with light gardening at around 11 a.m., and then he used a big hammer to break up some concrete. During that extreme effort, he felt chest pain.

As the pain became stronger, he was transferred by emergency service to the nearest hospital at 1 p.m. The ECG showed extreme ST elevation in anterior precordial leads (V1–6, D1, and AVL), and intravenous thrombolytic therapy was started (1.5 million units IV of streptokinase). Although chest pain diminished and ST elevation regressed from an initial 6 to 3 mm, (slide 6, Figure 6) the troponin and creatine phosphokinase (CK) values were high (>50 μmol/l and 3540 IU/l, respectively), so the physician in charge contacted our catheterization laboratory, and the patient was transferred by ambulance crew to our hospital.

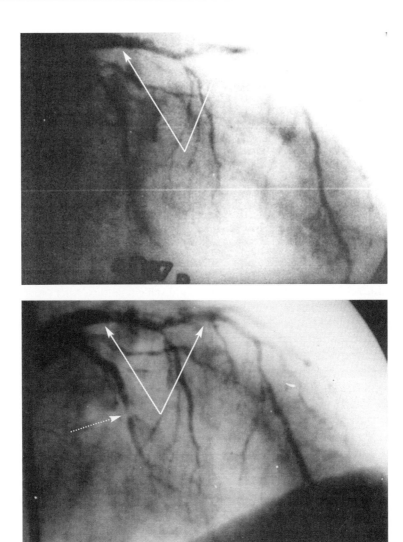

Figure 3   Left coronary artery angiography before PCI. October 24 2002. Solid arrows, lesion on LAD; dotted arrow, lesion on Cx

Coronary angiography was performed at 3 p.m. The LAD was widely patent, without visible thrombus or in-stent restenosis (slide 7, Figure 7), but with somewhat diminished flow; thrombotic occlusion of the Cypher stent therefore was presumed as the most probable cause of acute myocardial infarction. Restenosis at the site of POBA at the circumflex was also noted. No intervention was performed, and the

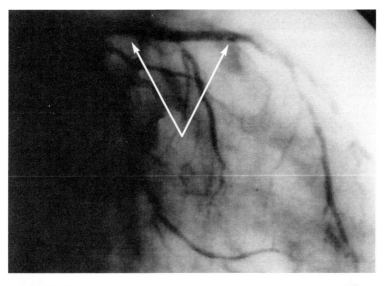

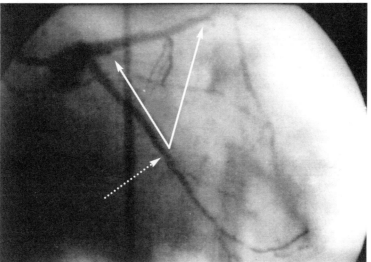

Figure 4   The final result of PCI. October 24 2002. Solid arrows, edges of Cypher 3.0 × 33 mm stent at 16 atm in LAD; dotted arrow, lesion on Cx after POBA 3.0 × 20 mm balloon at 12 atm

patient was transferred to the CCU for further treatment. As we did not have IIb/IIIa GP antagonist at our disposal, only the intravenous infusion of heparin was continued, together with long-acting mononitrate, metoprolol, aspirin, ticlopidine, sedatives, and atorvastatin. At 7 p.m., despite the adequate aPTT (98 sec), he had the

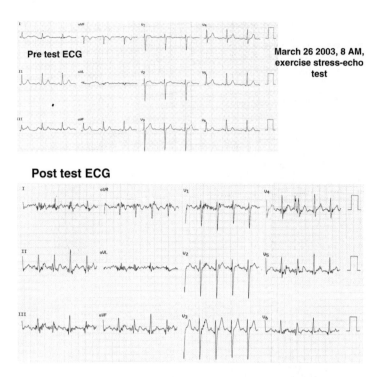

Figure 5   ECG before and immediately after exercise stress-echo test. March 26 2003, 8 a.m.

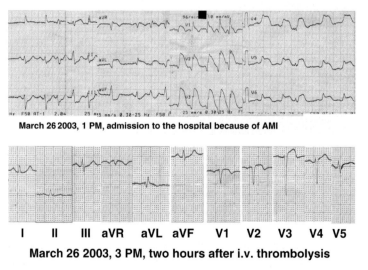

Figure 6   ECG at hospital admission because of AMI and two hours after initiation of i.v. thrombolysis

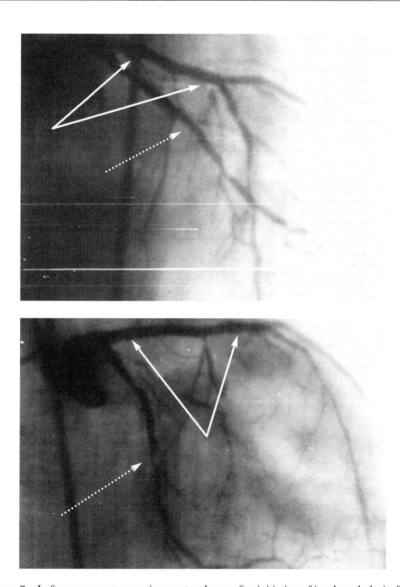

Figure 7 Left coronary artery angiogram two hours after initiation of i.v. thrombolysis. Solid arrows, edges of Cypher stent in LAD; dotted arrow, restenotic lesion on Cx at the site of POBA

reoccurrence of chest pain, with hemodynamic deterioration, worsening of ST segment elevation in precordial leads, hypotension, and repetitive ventricular fibrillations not responsive on multiple DC shocks; and he passed away at 7.45 p.m. The autopsy was canceled at the request of the family, according to the valid state law.

Lessons to be learned

1. Stent thrombosis on the LAD without intimal hyperplasia (restenosis), not restenotic lesion on the circumflex, was a cause of the fatal event.
2. Prothrombotic milieu can be so strong that reoccurrence of thrombosis after successful thrombolytic therapy could be triggered. So in retrospect, IIb/IIIa GP antagonist seems to be mandatory in such patients.
3. Exercise stress-echo test may well be the triggering factor for stent thrombosis at the site of DES implantation, particularly in the patients with complex lesions, even with double antiplatelet therapy. This possibility should be considered seriously, or alternatively the contrary proven.
4. The decision to perform stress-echo testing (exercise or pharmacological) in patients with DES should be made in each individual patient by weighing the pro and contra arguments depending on the expected information from the test.

REFERENCES

1. Gruntzig AR, Senning A, Siegenthaler WE. Nonoperative dilatation of coronary-artery stenosis: percutaneous transluminal coronary angioplasty. N Engl J Med 1979; 301: 61–68
2. Labovitz AJ, Kern MJ, et al. The effects of successful PTCA on left ventricular function: assessment by exercise echocardiography. Am Heart J 1989; 117: 1003–8
3. Massa D, Pirelli S, Gara E, et al. Exercise testing and dipyridamole echocardiography test before and 48 h after successful coronary angioplasty: prognostic implications. Eur Heart J 1989; 10 (Suppl G): 13–17
4. Picano E, Pirelli S, Marzilli M, et al. Usefulness of high-dose dipyridamole echocardiography test in coronary angioplasty. Circulation 1989; 80(4): 807–15
5. Broderick T, Sawada S, Armstrong WF, et al. Improvement in rest and exercise-induced wall motion abnormalities after coronary angioplasty: an exercise echocardiographic study. J Am Coll Cardiol 1990; 15(3): 591–9
6. Aboul-Enein H, Bengston JR, Adams DB, et al. Effect of the degree of effort on exercise echocardiography for the detection of restenosis after coronary artery angioplasty. Am Heart J 1991; 122(2): 430–7
7. Pirelli S, Danzi GB, Alberti A, et al. Comparison of usefulness of high-dose dipyridamole echocardiography and exercise electrocardiography for detection of asymptomatic restenosis after coronary angioplasty. Am J Cardiol 1991; 67(16): 1335–8
8. Pirelli S, Massa D, Faletra F, et al. Exercise electrocardiography versus dipyridamole echocardiography testing in coronary angioplasty. Early functional evaluation and prediction of angina recurrence. Circulation 1991; 83(Suppl 5): III38–42
9. McNeill AJ, Fioretti PM, el-Said SM, et al. Dobutamine stress echocardiography before and after coronary angioplasty. Am J Cardiol 1992; 69(8): 740–5
10. Akosah KO, Porter TR, Simon R, et al. Ischemia-induced regional wall motion abnormality is improved after coronary angioplasty: demonstration by dobutamine stress echocardiography. J Am Coll Cardiol 1993; 21(3): 584–9

11. Mertes H, Erbel R, Nixdorff U, et al. Exercise echocardiography for the evaluation of patients after nonsurgical coronary artery revascularization. J Am Coll Cardiol 1993; 21(5): 1087–93

12. Dagianti A, Rosanio S, Penco M, et al. Clinical and prognostic usefulness of supine bicycle exercise echocardiography in the functional evaluation of patients undergoing elective percutaneous transluminal coronary angioplasty. Circulation 1997; 95(5): 1176–84

13. Pirelli S, Danzi GB, Massa D, et al. Exercise thallium scintigraphy versus high-dose dipyridamole echocardiography testing for detection of asymptomatic restenosis in patients with positive exercise tests after coronary angioplasty. Am J Cardiol 1993; 71(12): 1052–6

14. Hecht HS, DeBord L, Shaw R, et al. Usefulness of supine bicycle stress echocardiography for detection of restenosis after percutaneous transluminal coronary angioplasty. Am J Cardiol 1993; 71(4): 293–6

15. Picano E, Sicari R. Special subsets of angiographically defined patients. In Picano E, ed. Stress echocardiography. New York: Springer Verlag 2003: 329–35

16. Ostojic M, Picano E, Stepanovic J, et al. Dipyridamole-exercise echocardiography test as a tool to assess physiologic benefit of percutaneous transluminal coronary angioplasty and directional coronary atherectomy in one-vessel coronary artery disease. Isr J Med Sci 1996; 32(10): 990

17. Ostojic M, Picano E, Beleslin B, et al. Dipyridamole-dobutamine echocardiography: a novel test for the detection of milder forms of coronary artery disease. J Am Coll Cardiol 1994; 23(5): 1115–22

18. Beleslin BD, Ostojic M, Stepanovic J, et al. Stress echocardiography in the detection of myocardial ischemia. Head-to-head comparison of exercise, dobutamine, and dipyridamole tests. Circulation 1994; 90(3): 1168–76

19. Miller DD, Verani MS. Current status of myocardial perfusion imaging after percutaneous transluminal coronary angioplasty. J Am Coll Cardiol 1994; 24(1): 260–6

20. Picano E, Palinkas A, Amyot R. Diagnosis of myocardial ischemia in hypertensive patients. J Hypertens 2001; 19: 1177–1183

21. Picano E. Stress echocardiography: a historical perspective. Am J Med 2003; 114(2): 126–30

22. Nedeljkovic MA, Ostojic M, Beleslin B, et al. Dipyridamole-atropine-induced myocardial infarction in a patient with patent epicardial coronary arteries. Herz 2001; 26(7): 485–8

23. Parodi G, Antoniucci D. Late coronary stent thrombosis associated with exercise testing. Catheter Cardiovasc Interv 2004; 61(4): 515–7

24. Maraj R, Fraifeld M, Owen, AN, et al. Coronary dissection and thrombosis associated with exercise testing three months after successful coronary stenting. Clin Cardiol 1999; 22(6): 426–8

25. Dash H. Delayed coronary occlusion after successful percutaneous transluminal coronary angioplasty: association with exercise testing. Am J Cardiol 1983; 52(8): 1143–4

26. Roffi M., Wenaweser P, Windecker S, et al. Early exercise after coronary stenting is safe. J Am Coll Cardiol 2003; 42(9): 1569–73

27. Waksman R, Ajani AE, White RL, et al. Prolonged antiplatelet therapy to prevent late thrombosis after intracoronary gamma-radiation in patients with in-stent restenosis: Washington Radiation for In-Stent Restenosis Trial plus 6 months of clopidogrel (WRIST PLUS). Circulation 2001; 103(19): 2332–5

28. Liistro F, Colombo A. Late acute thrombosis after paclitaxel eluting stent implantation. Heart 2001; 86(3): 262–4
29. Virmani RM, Guagliumi G, Farb A, et al. Localized hypersensitivity and late coronary thrombosis secondary to a sirolimus-eluting stent. Circulation 2004; 109: 701–5
30. Cutlip DE, Baim DS, Ho KK, et al. Stent thrombosis in the modern era: a pooled analysis of multicenter coronary stent clinical trials. Circulation 2001; 103(15): 1967–71
31. Meurin P, Domniez T, Bourmayan C. Coronary stent occlusion following strenuous exertion: is the risk actual? Is it preventable? Int J Cardiol 2000: 74(2–3): 249–51
32. Uren NG, Schwarzacher SP, Metz JA, et al. Predictors and outcomes of stent thrombosis: an intravascular ultrasound registry. Eur Heart J 2002; 23(2): 124–32
33. Wang F, Stouffer GA, Waxman S, Uretsky BF. Late coronary stent thrombosis: early vs. late stent thrombosis in the stent era. Catheter Cardiovasc Interv 2002; 55(2): 142–7
34. Kestin AS, Ellis PA, Barnard MR, et al. Effect of strenuous exercise on platelet activation state and reactivity. Circulation 1993; 88(4 Pt 1): 1502–11
35. Gibbons RJ, Balady GJ, Beasley JW, et al. ACC/AHA Guidelines for Exercise Testing. A report of the American College of Cardiology/American Heart Association Task Force on Practice Guidelines (Committee on Exercise Testing). J Am Coll Cardiol 1997; 30(1): 260–311
36. Picano E, Mathias WJ, Pingitore A, et al. Safety and tolerability of dobutamine-atropine stress echocardiography: a prospective, large scale, multicenter trial. Lancet 1994; 344: 1190–1192
37. Picano E, Marini C, Pirelli S, et al. Safety of intravenous high-dose dipyridamole echocardiography. The Echo-Persantine International Cooperative Study Group. Am J Cardiol 1992; 70(2): 252–8
38. Galloway MT, Paglieroni TG, Wun T, et al. Platelet activation during dobutamine stress echocardiography. Am Heart J 1995; 135: 888–900
39. Smith J. Effects of strenuous exercise on haemostasis. Br J Sports Med 2003; 37: 433–5

10

Cost–Effectiveness Analysis

Economic considerations of drug-eluting stents

Dan Greenberg PhD, *David J Cohen* MD, MSc

INTRODUCTION

Over the past decade, coronary stenting has emerged as the dominant form of percutaneous coronary revascularization. Bare-metal stents remain limited by a high incidence of restenosis, however, leading to frequent repeat revascularization procedures and substantial economic burden. Anti-proliferative drug-eluting stents (DES) represent one of the most innovative developments in interventional cardiology today, and studies involving several different stent platforms and anti-proliferative drug coatings have recently demonstrated dramatic reductions in restenosis rates compared with conventional bare-metal stents.[1-6] Although the clinical benefits of DES are increasingly evident, important concerns about their costs have been raised.[7] In this chapter, we summarize the current evidence on the economic impact of restenosis and explore the potential benefits and economic outcomes of DES. In addition to examining the long-term costs of this promising technology, we consider the potential cost-effectiveness of DES from a US healthcare system perspective and the impact of specific patient and lesion characteristics on these parameters.

CLINICAL AND ECONOMIC BURDEN OF RESTENOSIS

In order to understand fully the economic burden of coronary restenosis, we must investigate both the frequency of clinically important restenosis, the additional medical-care costs associated with diagnosis and treatment of restenosis, and the overall impact of restenosis on both the quality of life and long-term survival.

Direct medical-care costs of treating coronary restenosis

Most data regarding the impact of restenosis on long-term costs after PCI are derived from clinical trials[8-11] or from single-center series.[12] Although these studies may not

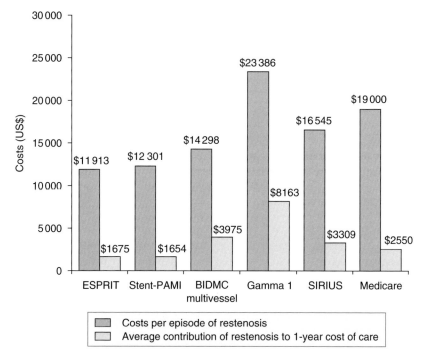

Figure 1 Average costs associated with the treatment of restenosis in selected stent populations, and the average added cost per patient during the first year after stent implantation.[40] BIDMC, Beth Israel-Deaconess Medical Center; ESPRIT, Enhanced Suppression of the Platelet IIb/IIIa Receptor with Integrilin Therapy; SIRIUS, SIRollimus-eluting stent in *de novo* coronary lesions; Stent-PAMI, Stent Primary Angioplasty in Myocardial Infarction

be applicable to the entire population of patients undergoing PCI, they nonetheless provide several important insights. For example, in the Enhanced Suppression of the Platelet IIb/IIIa Receptor with Integrilin Therapy (ESPRIT) trial, the mean cost for an admission to treat clinical restenosis was US$11 913 (compared with US$10 430 for an index hospitalization). On a population basis, restenosis added an average of US$1675 to each patient's cost of care during the first year after coronary stenting.[11] This value may be regarded as the direct 'economic burden' of restenosis in the ESPRIT trial population. Similar findings were noted in the Stent-Primary Angioplasty for Acute Myocardial Infarction (Stent-PAMI) trial of patients with acute myocardial infarction.[9] However, higher costs for each episode of clinical restenosis and higher economic burdens were noted in several distinct populations, including patients with in-stent restenosis undergoing treatment in the Gamma-1 trial[13] and patients undergoing multivessel PCI[12] (Figure 1). These diverse studies demonstrate that just as there is no single 'restenosis rate' for all patients who undergo PCI, there is no single cost or economic burden of restenosis; these values vary substantially according to the specific patient population under investigation.

We recently undertook a series of studies in an effort to determine the cost and economic burden of restenosis in the 'real world' of the US Medicare program. In this population, we found that the incidence of repeat revascularization between 1 month and 1 year after initial PCI was ~16%.[14] When one considers that ~15% of repeat revascularization procedures during the first year after PCI are related to treatment of other coronary lesions and not restenosis,[15,16] these population-based data indicate that the 'real-world' clinical restenosis rate in contemporary PCI is ~14%. It should be noted that this rate is approximately two-thirds of the rate seen in many clinical trials, because these trials frequently incorporate mandatory follow-up coronary angiography, which increases apparent clinical restenosis rates by up to 50%.[17,18] In the Medicare population, we calculated that the direct 1-year cost of repeat revascularization was ~US\$19 000 per episode, and the per capita economic burden of restenosis was ~US\$2500 per PCI patient.[14]

DO DRUG-ELUTING STENTS SAVE LIVES?

To date, no studies have demonstrated a convincing link between restenosis and either short- or long-term mortality. Unlike patients with *de novo* lesions, where plaque rupture and local thrombus formation may lead to acute myocardial infarction and death, clinically significant coronary restenosis is the result of progressive luminal renarrowing due to neointimal hyperplasia and vascular remodeling, and generally presents as a gradual recurrence of anginal symptoms and only rarely results in myocardial infarction.

Several lines of clinical evidence confirm the generally benign prognosis of coronary restenosis. Although rates of repeat revascularization following PTCA are five- to ten-fold higher than after bypass surgery, most randomized clinical trials have failed to demonstrate differences in long-term survival between these alternative forms of revascularization.[19–23] Moreover, in a study of more than 3300 patients who underwent angiographic restudy after PTCA, Weintraub and colleagues failed to identify any difference in six-year mortality between patients with and without restenosis.[24] Taken together, these data confirm the generally benign prognosis of coronary restenosis and suggest that even dramatic reductions in restenosis by DES are unlikely to improve substantially the long-term survival for patients undergoing PCI.

DO DRUG-ELUTING STENTS IMPROVE PATIENTS' HEALTH-RELATED QUALITY OF LIFE?

Numerous studies have documented the impact of restenosis on health-related quality of life (HRQOL). In the Optimum PTCA compared with Routine Stent Strategy (OPUS I) trial, evaluation of disease specific quality of life (as assessed by the

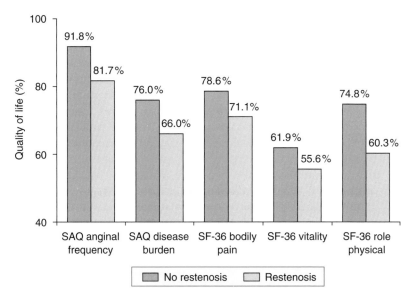

Figure 2   Quality of life of patients in the Stent-Primary Angioplasty for Acute Myocardial Infarction (Stent-PAMI) trial according to the occurrence of clinical restenosis (i.e. target-vessel revascularization) during follow-up.[26] At the 6-month follow-up, patients with no restenosis had significantly higher scores on the anginal frequency and disease-burden sub-scales of the Seattle Angina Questionnaire (SAQ), and higher scores on the bodily pain, role physical, and vitality scales of the SF-36 questionnaire. (Higher scores represent better quality of life/improved function)

Seattle Angina Questionnaire) demonstrated that patients without restenosis had less frequent angina, fewer physical limitations, and improved quality of life, compared with patients with restenosis.[25] Moreover, in a prospective quality-of-life substudy of the Stent-PAMI trial, Rinfret *et al.* found that compared with conventional balloon angioplasty, initial stenting was associated with significantly better HRQOL at the 6-month follow-up (Figure 2).[26] These differences were explained primarily by the reduced rates of angiographic and clinical restenosis associated with stenting in this trial. Although no studies to date have directly compared quality of life between patients receiving DES and conventional stents, it is nonetheless reasonable to assume that the lower rates of clinical restenosis and repeat interventions in patients treated with DES would have a positive impact on their HRQOL.

EVALUATING THE COST-EFFECTIVENESS OF TREATMENTS THAT REDUCE RESTENOSIS

In order to assess the economic value of any new medical technology, it is essential that the new technology be compared against the current standard of care.[27]

Cost-effectiveness analysis is a method for comparing the expected benefits of a medical technology with the net cost of the technology.[28] This relationship is expressed in terms of an *incremental cost-effectiveness ratio*, which is calculated by dividing the net cost of the treatment being evaluated (relative to standard of care), by its net benefits (also compared with standard of care):

$$\text{Incremental cost-effectiveness ratio} = \frac{\text{Cost}_{New} - \text{Cost}_{Standard}}{\text{Effectiveness}_{New} - \text{Effectiveness}_{Standard}}$$

In general, costs are measured in monetary terms, while any valued clinical outcome may be used to measure health benefits. Although any clinically relevant outcome measure can be used, the standard approach is to assess long-term health outcomes in terms of quality-adjusted life years (QALYs). The QALY concept uses years of life in perfect health as a common metric to value both life expectancy and quality of life. QALYs are calculated by weighting each time-interval in a given state of health by its 'utility' – a value between 0 and 1 that reflects the individual's preference for that health-state relative to perfect health (utility = 1) and death (utility = 0).[28] Once a cost-effectiveness ratio is calculated, it is typically compared with cost-effectiveness ratios for other therapies in a 'league table'. The threshold for determining whether a therapy is economically attractive varies with the available healthcare budget. In the USA, for example, cost-effectiveness ratios < US\$50 000 per QALY gained are viewed as favorable, and cost-effectiveness ratios between US\$50 000 and US\$100 000 per QALY gained are frequently considered to be in a 'gray zone'. In contrast, a cost-effectiveness ratio > US\$100 000 per QALY saved is viewed as economically unattractive in virtually all healthcare systems (including in the USA).[29]

Although the use of QALYs as an outcome measure in cost-effectiveness analysis is widely accepted, several pragmatic issues limit the attractiveness of this endpoint for valuing treatments whose principal benefit is preventing restenosis after PCI. Since there is no evidence that restenosis affects survival, one would not expect treatments whose sole benefit is a reduction in restenosis (such as DES) to improve population-level life expectancy. Although it is well-recognized that restenosis is associated with impaired QOL,[25,26,30] empirical data as to the overall impact of restenosis on quality-adjusted life expectancy are limited.

Given these limitations, several recent studies have used a disease-specific cost-effectiveness ratio: cost per repeat revascularization avoided.[9,13,17] The advantages of this endpoint are that it is simple to measure, can be easily integrated into standard data collection for clinical trials or registries, and is readily interpreted by both clinicians and patients. The primary limitation of this endpoint is that it is specific to the field of coronary revascularization and cannot be compared with cost-effectiveness ratios for other conditions, or against cost-effectiveness analyses using different outcome measures. Thus, determination of an appropriate cost-effectiveness threshold may be challenging.

Table 1   Evaluation of the cost-effectiveness of a treatment that reduces restenosis

---

Cost per quality-adjusted life year (QALY) gained
- Standard metric for cost-effectiveness analysis
- Allows comparison across different diseases (using a league table)
- Cost-effectiveness thresholds (i.e. societal willingness to pay for life-year gained) are reasonably defined

Cost per repeat revascularization avoided
- Readily measured in both clinical trials and observational studies
- Interpretable to both patients and clinicians

Within a specific healthcare system, however, comparison with other established (and reimbursed) technologies that can prevent coronary restenosis may serve as a useful benchmark. For example, within the US healthcare system, several technologies with cost-effectiveness ratios < US$10 000 per repeat revascularization avoided (e.g. brachytherapy for in-stent restenosis, elective coronary stenting vs. balloon angioplasty) have been widely adopted and are currently reimbursed by most third-party payers.[9,17] These observations thus suggest that therapies with cost-effectiveness ratios < US$10 000 per repeat revascularization avoided may be considered reasonably attractive within the US healthcare system. The evaluation of the cost-effectiveness of a treatment that reduces restenosis is summarized in Table 1.

ARE DES COST-EFFECTIVE (AND FOR WHICH PATIENTS)?

The procedural cost of PCI with DES is higher than for other PCI procedures, primarily due to the additional cost of the DES itself. However, use of DES is not expected to change the other cost components of PCI (i.e. diagnostic tests, complication rates, and hospital length of stay). Total treatment costs (initial and follow-up costs) will depend on the cost-offsets associated with reduced restenosis rates and reduction in the need for repeat revascularization procedures. However, given current levels of DES efficacy (75–80% relative risk reductions of restenosis), and DES costs (incremental cost of ~US$2000 per stent compared with bare-metal stents), it is unlikely that the long-term cost savings would fully offset the higher costs of DES themselves. Thus, the decision to adopt DES into clinical practice must consider whether the benefits of this technology are 'worth the costs'.

Evidence on the cost-effectiveness of DES can be provided from economic analyses alongside clinical trials, as well as disease-simulation models. To date, prospective economic analyses have been conducted alongside two randomized clinical trials comparing DES with BMS. The first such study was performed in conjunction with the RAVEL trial.[8] The economic analysis was based on resource utilization from the trial and unit costs from The Netherlands, and assumed a cost

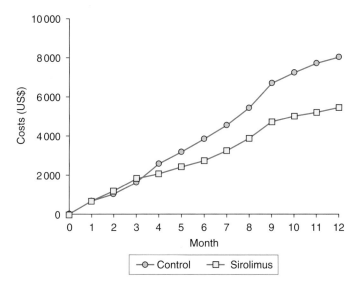

Figure 3   Results from the SIRIUS trial cost-effectiveness analysis.[10] While there was no difference in follow-up costs between the sirolimus stent and control arm during the first 3 months after the initial PCI, follow-up costs were substantially higher for the control arm at 12 months. This cost difference was due mainly to a reduced requirement for repeat revascularization procedures in the sirolimus-eluting stent arm

of €2000 for each sirolimus-eluting stent. In RAVEL, the initial procedural costs were €1284 higher for patients treated with DES, but reductions in follow-up costs offset most of the additional expenses. As a result, at the 12-month follow-up, the sirolimus-eluting stent was associated with an additional cost of only €166 per patient.

More recently, we reported preliminary results from a prospective economic evaluation performed in conjunction with the US SIRIUS trial.[10] For this study, costs were assessed from a US healthcare system perspective over a one-year time horizon. Based on current national averages, we assumed that each DES would cost US$2700 and each BMS would cost US$700. Initial hospital costs were approximately US$2800 higher with the sirolimus-eluting stent compared with the bare-metal stent (US$11 345 vs. US$8464, $p < 0.001$). However, much of this difference in initial costs was offset by lower follow-up costs (US$5468 vs. US$8040, $p < 0.001$), mainly due to a reduced requirement for repeat revascularization procedures (Figure 3). Thus, at 12 months, the DES strategy cost an average of US$309/patient more than the BMS strategy, yielding cost-effectiveness ratios of US$1650 per repeat revascularization avoided and US$27 500 per QALY gained.

It is important to recognize that the results of these trial-based economic studies cannot necessarily be extrapolated to the conditions of routine clinical practice. For example, although both studies incorporated adjustments or event adjudication to limit the extent to which protocol-driven costs affected the economic outcomes, it is difficult to account fully for the impact of the 'oculostenotic reflex' on clinical outcomes in trials that incorporate routine angiographic follow-up. Moreover, patients enrolled in clinical trials are highly selected and are often treated in high-volume medical centers, thus limiting the generalizability of trial results.

To overcome these limitations, we have developed a decision-analysis model to evaluate the cost-effectiveness of DES for patients undergoing single-vessel PCI.[31,32] The model's perspective is that of the US healthcare system. Data for the model were derived from a database that currently contains one-year outcomes on more than 6000 patients undergoing PCI with conventional stent implantation.[16] Costs for revascularization procedures, their associated complications, and treatment of restenosis were based on pooled economic data from several multicenter trials of contemporary PCI involving more than 3000 patients.[31] Key assumptions of the model were based, as far as possible, on empirically derived data; key assumptions included an average target-vessel revascularization (TVR) rate for BMS of 14%,[14,16,33] an 80% reduction in TVR with DES,[1,34] an incremental cost of US$2000 per DES, and a mean utilization of 1.3 stents per *single-vessel* stent procedure.[35]

Over a two-year follow-up period, this model projected that overall medical care costs with DES would be ~US$900/patient higher than with bare-metal stents, with an incremental cost-effectiveness ratio of ~US$7000 per repeat revascularization avoided. Sensitivity analyses demonstrated that treatment with DES would be cost-saving for patients with a BMS TVR rate > 20% and cost-effective (i.e. cost-effectiveness ratio < US$10 000/repeat revascularization avoided) for patients with a BMS TVR rate > 12% (Figure 4).

Further insight into the ideal patient population for implantation of DES may be derived from statistical models to predict restenosis after BMS implantation. Most studies have identified smaller reference-vessel diameter, greater lesion length, and the presence of diabetes as consistent predictors of both angiographic and clinical restenosis after conventional stent implantation.[16,36] By combining these predicted restenosis rates with the previously described cost-effectiveness model, it is possible to estimate the cost-effectiveness of DES for a variety of specific patient and lesion characteristics. This approach demonstrates that compared with conventional stents, DES would be cost-saving for only a modest proportion of the current PCI population. On the other hand, these models also indicate that DES should be *economically attractive* (i.e. cost-effectiveness ratio < US$10 000 per repeat revascularization avoided) for virtually all diabetic patients and for nondiabetic patients with smaller vessels (reference-vessel diameter < 3.0 mm) and longer lesions (lesion length > 15 mm)[37].

Several other studies in Europe have examined the economic impact of DES using decision-analysis models and budget-impact analyses. Lamotte *et al.*[38] used a decision-analysis model to assess the cost-effectiveness of sirolimus-eluting stents (estimated cost €2300/stent) for treatment of single-vessel coronary disease from the perspective of the Belgian healthcare system. They found that the incremental cost-effectiveness ratio of the sirolimus-eluting stent compared with a bare-metal stent at

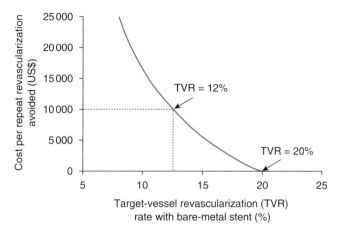

Figure 4   Relationship between the TVR rate with BMS implantation and the incremental cost-effectiveness of DES implantation for patients undergoing single-vessel PCI. This analysis assumes an incremental cost of US$2000 per DES, an average utilization of 1.3 stents per procedure, and a reduction by DES of the TVR rate by 80% compared with BMS. The model projects that DES implantation will be reasonably cost-effective (i.e. cost-effectiveness ratio < US$10 000 per repeat revascularization avoided) for patients with an expected BMS TVR rate > 12%; cost-savings, are projected for patients with TVR rates > 20%[37]

1 year varied from €1119 to €2947 per repeat revascularization avoided and depended primarily on the vessel size and lesion length. A second decision model used average charges for the Italian national healthcare system to estimate the overall budget impact of DES for treating patients with single-vessel or multivessel disease.[39] In the first year after revascularization, use of drug-eluting stents was projected to prevent 123–182 revascularizations per 1000 patients compared with conventional stenting and resulted in net savings of €1036–€1800 per treated patient. The overall annual savings to the Italian system were estimated to be about €39 million.

INTERPRETING FINDINGS FROM ECONOMIC ANALYSES

The findings from these economic analyses should be interpreted with caution however, particularly with respect to the underlying patient population and relevant healthcare system. For example, PCI costs are highly influenced by resource utilization in the catheterization laboratory, and particularly by the number of stents used per procedure. These patterns may differ substantially among practitioners, institutions, and healthcare systems. Thus, differences in both medical practices and costs in different healthcare systems make international comparisons difficult.

    A further limitation of the available economic analyses is their focus on direct medical costs (i.e. repeat procedures, hospital admissions, diagnostic tests, and medication use). Although coronary restenosis has a relatively short-lived impact on quality of life, it may also be associated with indirect costs such as productivity losses on the part of both patients and care-givers. Inclusion of these costs in an economic analysis would make the use of DES even more economically attractive than current studies suggest.

Finally, it is important to recognize that the available data on both the efficacy and cost-effectiveness of DES are based almost entirely on studies of relatively ideal candidates for this technology. In routine clinical practice, there will undoubtedly be important differences in the underlying clinical and angiographic characteristics, and these differences may have important effects on both treatment efficacy (i.e. relative risk reduction in TVR rates) as well as treatment costs (e.g. because of greater utilization of multiple stents to treat more diffuse lesions and multivessel disease). The ultimate cost-effectiveness of this promising technology will depend on the complex interplay of these factors and cannot be predicted with certainty at the present time. Moreover, as competitive devices enter the DES market, it is likely that the price of DES will fall. Although the effect of falling stent prices will certainly improve the cost-effectiveness of DES relative to BMS, it is difficult to predict either the timing or rate of these key developments.

ALTERNATIVE PERSPECTIVES

The preceding discussion focused on the economic impact of DES from a health-care-system perspective. When considering the overall economic impact of DES, however, it is important to recognize that alternative perspectives may be more relevant to different stakeholders. From the hospital perspective, the profitability of DES procedures depends on third-party reimbursement and the cost of the stent. Currently, in the US private healthcare system, insufficient third-party reimbursement for DES procedures may result in financial loss to the hospital. Moreover, given the benefits of DES in reducing restenosis, hospitals will face further loss of revenue due to the expected downstream reduction in the need for repeat revascularization procedures. Finally, and most importantly, US hospitals will face a loss of revenue due to the expected substitution of less-remunerative DES procedures for bypass surgery – a highly lucrative and profitable procedure for many hospitals.

CONCLUSIONS

The development of drug-eluting coronary stents has been hailed as a true breakthrough in interventional cardiology. Although the use of DES is unlikely to reduce already low rates of in-hospital death and acute myocardial infarction in patients receiving PCI, substantial reductions in restenosis and repeat revascularization should be apparent within the first 6–12 months after their introduction. The overall budget impact of DES is difficult to predict. It will depend on a variety of factors including the overall adoption rate, the target population that receives DES, device costs, clinical effectiveness in the 'real world', and conversion rates from bypass surgery to PCI. Even if DES are cost-effective compared with standard PCI, however, they may not be readily adopted worldwide as the new standard-of-care until appropriate budgets and reimbursement levels are in place to cover fully the higher initial treatment costs.

Currently there is no single answer to the question: 'Are drug-eluting stents cost-effective?' The cost-effectiveness of DES depends on the target population and the specific treatment under comparison (e.g. bare-metal stenting, bypass surgery, or medical therapy), as well as on the perspective of the analysis. Nonetheless, at least for the patient population currently undergoing PCI in the USA, simulation models as well as prospective analyses from clinical trials suggest that DES will be reasonably cost-effective for the majority of patients, and even cost saving for a large subgroup of patients who are at relatively high risk of clinical restenosis with conventional PCI techniques. In the future, lower incremental costs for DES should render this technology cost-saving for a much larger subgroup of PCI patients and broaden the ideal target population.

REFERENCES

1. Morice MC, Serruys PW, Sousa JE, et al. A randomized comparison of a sirolimus-eluting stent with a standard stent for coronary revascularization. N Engl J Med 2002; 346: 1773–80
2. Moses JW, Leon MB, Popma JJ, et al. Sirolimus-eluting stents versus standard stents in patients with stenosis in a native coronary artery. N Engl J Med 2003; 349: 1315–23
3. Schofer J, Schluter M, Gershlick AH, et al. Sirolimus-eluting stents for treatment of patients with long atherosclerotic lesions in small coronary arteries: double-blind, randomised controlled trial (E-SIRIUS). Lancet 2003; 362: 1093–9
4. Grube E, Silber S, Hauptmann KE, et al. Taxus I: six- and twelve-month results from a randomized, double-blind trial on a slow-release paclitaxel-eluting stent for de novo coronary lesions. Circulation 2003; 107: 38–42
5. Park SJ, Shim WH, Ho DS, et al. A paclitaxel-eluting stent for the prevention of coronary restenosis. N Engl J Med 2003; 348: 1537–45
6. Stone GW, Ellis SG, Cox DA, et al. A polymer-based, paclitaxel-eluting stent in patients with coronary artery disease. N Engl J Med 2004; 350: 221–31
7. O'Neill WW, Leon MB. Drug-eluting stents: costs versus clinical benefit. Circulation 2003; 107: 3008–11
8. van Hout BA, Lindeboom WK, Morice MC, et al. Cost-effectiveness of the sirolimus eluting Bx-Velocity stent: 1-year results. Eur Heart J 2002; 23 (Suppl.): 691
9. Cohen DJ, Taira DA, Berezin R, et al. Cost-effectiveness of coronary stenting in acute myocardial infarction: results from the stent primary angioplasty in myocardial infarction (stent-PAMI) trial. Circulation 2001; 104: 3039–45
10. Cohen DJ, Bakhai A, Shi C, et al. Cost-effectiveness of sirolimus drug-eluting stents for the treatment of complex coronary stenoses: results from the randomized SIRIUS trial. J Am Coll Cardiol 2003; 41: 32A
11. Cohen DJ, Cosgrove RS, Berezin RH, et al. Cost-effectiveness of eptifibatide in patients undergoing planned coronary stenting. Results from the ESPRIT trial (abstract). Circulation 2001; 104: I-386–I-387

12. Reynolds MR, Neil N, Ho KK, et al. Clinical and economic outcomes of multivessel coronary stenting compared with bypass surgery: a single-center US experience. Am Heart J 2003; 145: 334–42

13. Cohen DJ, Cosgrove RS, Berezin RH, et al. Cost-effectiveness of gamma radiation for treatment of in-stent restenosis: results from the Gamma-1 trial. Circulation 2002; 106: 691–7

14. Clark MA, Bakhai A, Lacey M, et al. The clinical and economic burden of restenosis in the medicare population. Presented at 4th Scientific Forum on Quality of Care and Outcomes Research in Cardiovascular Disease and Stroke, Washington, DC, October 13–14, 2002. Circulation 2002; 106: 76e–123

15. Kimmel SE, Sauer WH, Brensinger C, et al. Relationship between coronary angioplasty laboratory volume and outcomes after hospital discharge. Am Heart J 2002; 143: 833–40

16. Cutlip DE, Chauhan MS, Baim DS, et al. Clinical restenosis after coronary stenting: perspectives from multicenter clinical trials. J Am Coll Cardiol 2002; 40: 2082–9

17. Serruys PW, van Hout B, Bonnier H, et al. Randomised comparison of implantation of heparin-coated stents with balloon angioplasty in selected patients with coronary artery disease (Benestent II). Lancet 1998; 352: 673–81

18. Baim DS, Cutlip DE, Midei M, et al. Final results of a randomized trial comparing the Multi-Link stent with the Palmaz-Schatz stent for narrowings in native coronary arteries. Am J Cardiol 2001; 87: 157–62

19. Legrand VM, Serruys PW, Unger F, et al. Three-year outcome after coronary stenting versus bypass surgery for the treatment of multivessel disease. Circulation 2004; 109: 1114–20

20. The Bypass Angioplasty Revascularization Investigation (BARI) Investigators. Comparison of coronary bypass surgery with angioplasty in patients with multivessel disease. N Engl J Med 1996; 335: 217–25

21. King SB 3rd, Kosinski AS, Guyton RA, et al. Eight-year mortality in the Emory Angioplasty versus Surgery Trial (EAST). J Am Coll Cardiol 2000; 35: 1116–21

22. Serruys PW, Unger F, Sousa JE, et al. Comparison of coronary-artery bypass surgery and stenting for the treatment of multivessel disease. N Engl J Med 2001; 344: 1117–24

23. Pocock SJ, Henderson RA, Rickards AF, et al. Meta-analysis of randomised trials comparing coronary angioplasty with bypass surgery. Lancet 1995; 346: 1184–9

24. Weintraub WS, Ghazzal ZM, Douglas JS Jr., et al. Long-term clinical follow-up in patients with angiographic restudy after successful angioplasty. Circulation 1993; 87: 831–40

25. Weaver WD, Reisman MA, Griffin JJ, et al. Optimum percutaneous transluminal coronary angioplasty compared with routine stent strategy trial (OPUS-1): a randomised trial. Lancet 2000; 355: 2199–203

26. Rinfret S, Grines CL, Cosgrove RS, et al. Quality of life after balloon angioplasty or stenting for acute myocardial infarction. One-year results from the Stent-PAMI trial. J Am Coll Cardiol 2001; 38: 1614–21

27. Gold M, Siegel J, Russel L, Weinstein M. Cost-effectiveness in health and medicine. New York: Oxford University Press, 1996

28. Weinstein MC, Stason WB. Foundations of cost-effectiveness analysis for health and medical practices. N Engl J Med 1977; 296: 716–21

29. Goldman L, Gordon DJ, Rifkind BM, et al. Cost and health implications of cholesterol lowering. Circulation 1992; 85: 1960–8

30. Serruys PW, de Jaegere P, Kiemeneij F, et al and BENESTENT Study Group. A comparison of balloon-expandable-stent implantation with balloon angioplasty in patients with coronary artery disease. N Engl J Med 1994; 331: 489–95
31. Greenberg D, Cohen DJ. Examining the economic impact of restenosis: implications for the cost-effectiveness of an antiproliferative stent. Z Kardiol 2002; 91: 137–43
32. Greenberg D, Bakhai A, Neil N, et al. Modeling the impact of patient and lesion characteristics on the cost-effectiveness of drug-eluting stents. J Am Coll Cardiol 2003; 41: 538A
33. Holmes DR, Jr., Savage M, LaBlanche JM, et al. Results of Prevention of REStenosis with Tranilast and its Outcomes (PRESTO) trial. Circulation 2002; 106: 1243–50
34. Moses JW, Leon MB, Popma JJ, et al. Sirolimus-eluting stents versus standard stents in patients with stenosis in a native coronary artery. N Engl J Med 2003; 349: 1315–23
35. Cohen DJ, O'Shea JC, Pacchiana CM, et al. In-hospital costs of coronary stent implantation with and without eptifibatide (the ESPRIT Trial). Enhanced Suppression of the Platelet IIb/IIIa Receptor with Integrilin. Am J Cardiol 2002; 89: 61–4
36. Serruys PW, Kay IP, Disco C, et al. Periprocedural quantitative coronary angiography after Palmaz-Schatz stent implantation predicts the restenosis rate at six months: results of a meta-analysis of the BElgian NEtherlands Stent study (BENESTENT) I, BENESTENT II Pilot, BENESTENT II and MUSIC Multicenter Ultrasound Stent In Coronaries trials. J Am Coll Cardiol 1999; 34: 1067–74
37. Greenberg D, Bakhai A, Cohen DJ. Can we afford to eliminate restenosis? Can we afford not to? J Am Coll Cardiol 2004; 43: 513–8
38. Lamotte M, Annemas L, De Jong P. Drug-eluting stents in coronary disease: assessments of outcomes and cost-effectiveness. Eur Heart J 2002; 23 (Suppl): 137
39. Marchetti M, Tarricone R, Lamotte M, et al. Cost-effectiveness and budget impact of the sirolimus-eluting stent in the stent area. Value Health 2002; 5: 457
40. Greenberg J, Bakhai A, Cohen DJ. Do the benefits of new technology outweigh the costs? The case of drug-eluting stents. Am J Drug Deliv 2003; 1: 255–266

Index